Coping wit

D0545910

DUDLEY PUBLIC LIBRARIES

with the
Society.
n clinical
a variety
ognitive
mitment
apy that
client(s).
ariety of
to living
oblems,
nditions
service
also has
rtments.
alth and

Council-
n-based
She is a
member
erapies,
d a team
erapists
pervisor
cal and
ultant at
ondon,
hools in
t in the
ing, the
ological

present these topics at conferences in the UK and abroad.

Professor Robert Bor is a director of Dynamic Change Consultants (www. dcclinical.com), and Lead Clinical Psychologist in Medical Specialties at the Royal Free Hospital, London. A chartered clinical, counselling and health psychologist registered with the Health and Care Professions Council, he is also a fellow of the British Psychological Society and a member of the American Psychological Association. He has over 30 years' experience consulting in clinical and organizational settings in the UK and abroad. A UKCP-registered family and couples therapist, having specialized in systemic therapy at the Tavistock Clinic, London, Rob also practises cognitive behavioural therapy and is an advocate of time-limited and solution-focused therapeutic approaches. He works with children, adolescents, adults, couples, families and teams within organizations, and is Consulting Psychologist to Leaders in Oncology Care and the London Clinic (both in Harley Street), and to St Paul's School, the Royal Ballet School and JFS in London. He also provides psychological consultations and executive coaching to organizations such as PwC and UBS, among others, in London and abroad. Rob is an accredited aviation psychologist and Honorary Civilian Psychologist to the Royal Air Force. He holds the Freedom of the City of London and is a Churchill Fellow.

Overcoming Common Problems

Coping with the Psychological Effects of Illness

Strategies to manage anxiety and depression

DR FRAN SMITH,
DR CARINA ERIKSEN
and
PROFESSOR ROBERT BOR

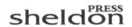

First published in Great Britain in 2015

Sheldon Press
36 Causton Street
London SW1P 4ST
www.sheldonpress.co.uk

The authors and publisher have made every effort to ensure that the external
website and email addresses included in this book are correct and up to date at the
time of going to press. The authors and publisher are not responsible for the content,
quality or continuing accessibility of the sites.

British Library Cataloguing-in-Publication Data
A catalogue record for this book is available from the British Library

ISBN 978–1–84709–343–1
eBook ISBN 978–1–84709–344–8

Typeset by Caroline Waldron, Wirral, Cheshire
First printed in Great Britain by Ashford Colour Press
Subsequently digitally reprinted in Great Britain

eBook by Fakenham Prepress Solutions, Fakenham, Norfolk NR21 8NN

Produced on paper from sustainable forests

Contents

1

Introduction and overview

Having a physical illness affects us psychologically in two main ways. On one level it is an individual matter that can affect how we think, behave and feel, both emotionally and physically. On another level it affects our relationships with people around us, our patterns of support and our life roles.

A health problem does not have the same effects on everyone. There are factors that influence how people react to, cope with and adjust to becoming unwell. In this book we will support you in gaining an understanding of the psychological effects of living with acute or chronic medical conditions and show you ways in which to adapt and cope better with the challenges.

Hardly a week goes by without some mention in the media of promising advances and breakthroughs in the treatment of certain medical conditions. Medical science in our generation has developed in unprecedented ways. Many cancers are treatable and some are even curable. HIV disease, which 30 years ago was almost inevitably fatal, can now be managed as a chronic, lifelong condition on an outpatient basis, theoretically affording a normal lifespan if diagnosis is made early and the treatment is well tolerated. These and many other examples of exciting and welcome developments in healthcare, however, do not always convey any sense of the psychological impact of this type of condition on those who must live with the disease.

Also, as mentioned above, these conditions have an impact not only on the individual but also on that person's family and other caregivers, and therefore the true psychological impact of chronic or acute health conditions ripples out far beyond just the one person.

Some medical advances arrive too late to benefit those who are already living with a particular health condition. For others the advances may be of limited benefit because of the costs of healthcare, the side effects of treatment, additional medical problems that may have developed as a consequence of the original condition and, in some circumstances, rationing in healthcare. Also, the fact that some of these advances are a result of laboratory studies but have not yet been proven in real-life situations means that, for practical purposes, the treatment may not yet be available to all patients.

Any medical condition can impose significant physical, emotional and practical challenges, but those which are regarded as acute (sudden onset) or chronic (long-developing) can be some of the hardest to bear. A diagnosis of a serious medical condition can wreak havoc in our lives and affect all aspects of our functioning and daily living. Work, recreation, relationships, routines, habits – and of course how we feel in ourselves – are all likely to be affected. As well as being life-changing, diagnosis of a medical problem can, in some cases, also signify that life itself is threatened.

Of course, every person's situation is unique, but in our professional experience the psychological effects of illness or chronic health conditions can be as hard to bear as the physical effects. This is not an overstatement – it rather reflects the results of several scientific studies of coping with illness, as well as our own clinical experience of working with people who have a broad spectrum of medical conditions. Most medical conditions in the acute and chronic categories also have a negative impact on self-confidence, mood, identity, capability, sleep and capacity for sexual intimacy or even functioning. These are just a few of the possible psychological effects which we discuss in this book.

Different health issues affect people in both obvious and unexpected ways. Exactly what effects they have will depend on your age and stage of life, your gender and your role in the family, past and current patterns of relationships within your family, the nature of your medical condition and how it affects you, your relationship with professionals such as doctors, nurses and other caregivers, and your ideas about and experiences of coping with being unwell, as well as personal circumstances such as your finances and home set-up.

Physical reactions to health problems cannot always be separated from psychological reactions. Certain conditions, or indeed the effects of the treatment of these conditions, can have profound and even scarring psychological consequences. The medical condition itself may, for example, cause you to be constantly tired, unable to sleep in spite of deep fatigue, in pain or suffering from itching, visual or auditory changes or discomfort, stomach problems such as constipation or diarrhoea with all the attendant embarrassment, inconvenience and restrictions, or difficulties with speech, attention span and everyday comprehension. These and many other effects may stem directly from your medical condition or from the treatment for that condition, and can on their own weigh you down psychologically.

We recognize that the challenges of illness can sometimes leave you feeling confused and overwhelmed. Your self-confidence may plummet and you may be emotionally upset. Each of these reactions can in turn affect your ability to cope. These challenges and physical symptoms may also affect relationship patterns with loved ones, with friends and indeed with professional caregivers. We have written this book with you and your experiences in mind. It is designed to help you cope better with your circumstances.

Our starting point is first to help you to develop an understanding of how acute or chronic illness can affect people. We highlight some specific and commonly occurring physical and emotional symptoms. Further on in the book we will focus on anxiety and depression, as these are arguably the two most commonly presenting psychological difficulties that people describe.

The book also addresses how to improve the support around you in the form of family and friends, and we extend this to dealing with your communication and relationship with professional caregivers as well.

We cannot hope, of course, to provide solutions to every problem you might encounter. However, with our extensive clinical and research experience we will share with you ways in which you can better understand and cope with some of the psychological effects of chronic and acute illness.

In the face of uncertainty about the course of your condition, for example, you might predominantly experience low mood and feelings of hopelessness, or perhaps struggle with worry and anxiety. In this book you will be encouraged to reflect on identifying your own unique presenting problems and responses to illness and to draw on the techniques and skills described in this book which are most relevant to you personally.

A message of hope

This book offers an empowering self-help approach derived from extensive current and evidence-based practice. It focuses on practical solutions to managing health conditions and coping with the experience of being unwell.

The book also focuses on living better with – and getting on top of – the emotionally challenging aspects of living with illness. We aim to convey a message of hope that, even when confronted with life-challenging situations and serious health difficulties, it is possible to approach your unique situation with greater confidence if you have appropriate knowledge, help and accessible social and professional support. This can alter the impact that your condition has on you, physically and emotionally, as well as on your relationships. We believe that better support improves health outcomes and we aim to arm you with strategies and techniques to improve your own coping.

So many of our clients with serious health conditions, chronic and acute, and those who work with our colleagues in countless clinical centres worldwide, report feeling that their illness has removed control from many aspects of their lives. Obviously this is a seriously unwelcome change for most people. However, by developing a clear and deep understanding of your psychological reactions, you can help yourself to regain a sense of control and take greater charge of your own care, your treatment, your coping and your emotions.

The course, treatment and medical outcome of your condition are not things you will always be able to control. You may find yourself relying on the input and intervention of medical specialists and other professionals. However, coping with a serious medical condition is as much about managing the psychological aspects as the practicalities, and of course it is the psychological factors which you can more directly influence through how you choose to live with your situation.

While it is necessary to trust in medical professionals to monitor, advise, assess and treat you, your psychological response is something *you* can work on yourself – and indeed is something that ultimately only you can do. Managing your thoughts and feelings can improve your mental health, and positive psychological responses have been clearly demonstrated to improve health outcomes, so this is something valuable that you can contribute to the successful management of your health condition.

Managing and improving your psychological response and wellbeing can be started on your own, in the context of family relationships and with the support of qualified professionals such as psychologists and counsellors. This book addresses how, in all these contexts, you can better understand and take charge of the way you cope psychologically.

Taking greater charge of your feelings and the management of your condition can be as simple as gaining the confidence to question your doctor about your treatment or possible side effects from some prescribed medications. It can also be as complex and sensitive as asking about the possible course of your condition, the likely outcome and, if the condition is untreatable, what may lie ahead for you and how best you can prepare for this. Taking charge of your health in this way can help you to regain a sense of control and mastery, rebuild your confidence and improve your wellbeing. It can also in some cases help you to overcome specific symptoms such as sleep or eating difficulties if, for example, these are linked to stress and worry.

Our approach

We aim to provide a practical and helpful handbook for people adapting to the emotional challenges of living with acute or chronic health conditions. Where possible we also point you towards other sources that can help.

This book draws primarily from cognitive behavioural therapy and mindfulness-based approaches. These are two of the most prominent and modern psychological approaches, particularly in the NHS and in time-limited therapy. We will now briefly outline these approaches.

Cognitive behavioural therapy

Cognitive behavioural therapy (CBT) is a modern, practical and evidence-based model. It has been shown to be effective when working with many psychological conditions and experiences, including adjusting to being unwell. The approach is upfront and practical, just as it is when we meet people face to face in counselling sessions. The model suggests that in any given situation there are four aspects dictating how you experience that situation.

1 *Thoughts* This is your mental activity, which is sometimes referred to as 'cognition'. What is going on in your mind? What are you focusing on? Where is your attention? It involves any images or stories your mind is telling you about the situation and includes memories, fantasies, worries, ideas, judgements, problem-solving and so on.
2 *Feelings* This is your emotional experience. Usually we can name our feelings using one word, such as 'happy', 'sad', 'angry', 'jealous', 'frightened'.
3 *Behaviour* This relates to what you are actually doing. If people were watching you, what would they see you doing? For example, are you looking up symptoms on the internet, calling friends for reassurance, lying in bed, going for a walk . . .?
4 *Body* This relates to how you are feeling physically. What is your physiological experience? Are you in pain? Are you hot or cold? Tired or agitated?

All these aspects are interconnected and all affect each other. For this reason you can develop patterns and cycles that can be self-perpetuating. Some of these patterns can be very unhelpful and can add considerably to any suffering that you are already experiencing, but the good news is that if you change one aspect of the cycle then the whole cycle changes. When you start to understand the cycles and where you tend to get stuck, you can plan how to change them and develop new and more helpful and adaptive patterns that reduce your overall experience of distress. Figure 1.1 illustrates the interactions between our thoughts, feelings, behaviour and body. We will draw on this diagram throughout the book to explain examples of common unhelpful patterns.

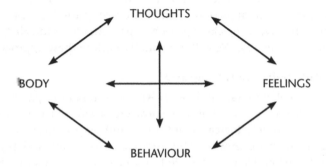

Figure 1.1 Interactions between our thoughts, feelings, behaviour and body

Mindfulness

In the last 20 years psychologists and other researchers and practitioners have been developing programmes in which people are taught mindfulness skills. These skills, which can be used to help cope with pain and suffering, help us respond differently to internal and external experiences, and there is evidence to show that they are effective.[1] Researchers have studied the efficacy of mindfulness skills in the management of chronic pain and the suffering and stress of illness. Indeed, they report that mindfulness meditation can be as effective as painkillers and can enhance nature's healing powers within the body. Mindfulness has also been shown to reduce significantly anxiety, depression, insomnia, irritability and fatigue that can come from chronic pain and illness.[2]

What is mindfulness?

Mindfulness is the opposite of 'automatic pilot mode'. Do you ever notice that you can be walking down a street but your mind feels a million miles away? You might be thinking about your appointment with your doctor tomorrow or an argument you had with your partner last night. Wherever your mind is, it is certainly not in the present moment. Many of us live most of our lives like this, with our attention focused on either the future or the past. And in the meantime we miss what is happening right now. Mindfulness is about being in the 'here and now'. Rather than 'doing' all the time, it is about 'being'. It is about letting go of our struggle with what has been or will be and accepting what is happening in this moment. It offers a helpful way of letting go of unhelpful patterns of thinking, feeling and behaving and has been shown to improve psychological wellbeing and resilience. In Chapter 4 we look at how mindfulness-based therapies are usefully applied to living with illness.

In addition to CBT and mindfulness approaches, our training and broad expertise means that we can bring together other established psychological techniques, such as systemic therapy, solution-focused therapy and acceptance and commitment therapy. We also draw on our solid base of clinical experience and use case vignettes to illustrate some of the shared experiences of people making their own adjustment to health conditions. We show the effectiveness of the interventions described and the unique solutions to their problems which people generate for themselves.

In this book we also try to avoid jargon and to be clear and direct in style. This is a simple rather than a simplistic approach – our aim is not to mystify and create a mystique, but to detail and explain a CBT approach to a serious subject in a straightforward way. Our aim is to help and educate, not to befuddle.

There is much debate about the language to use when referring to a range of physical health problems. Many health professionals now prefer the use of more inclusive and neutral language such as 'physical health conditions' rather than the word 'illness'. However, because this book is directed towards the general public, we have used the terminology most familiar to service users in the hope that the language will be commonplace and easily understood. For this reason the term 'illness' is used throughout the book.

We specifically avoid a 'one-size-fits-all' approach to therapy as every day we are reminded of the unique, particular and specific ways in which people cope with and adapt to life-challenging circumstances. This book is in no way prescriptive, because no one – and especially not a psychologist – should tell you how to live your life.

As we have already said, the main focus of this book is on the emotional effects of living with an acute or chronic health condition. We specifically do not address medical or clinical aspects of any particular condition, as these are best explored in your clinical visits with your health professionals. Medical problems are obviously never welcome, and a diagnosis of a serious health condition can be hard to bear. We hope that the ideas, information and psychological skills discussed in this book will help you and your loved ones to move forward and achieve a life which is fulfilling and positive in spite of the challenges you are currently facing.

The rest of the book

You can either go through the book from beginning to end or go directly to the sections which are most relevant to you, whatever you find most helpful. The book is set out as follows:

Chapter 1 – Introduction and overview

Chapter 2 – Typology of medical conditions

This chapter differentiates some key dimensions of illness, including the onset, course, outcome and degree of incapacitation, and considers the impact of these dimensions on the lives of people living with them.

Chapter 3 – What affects how we cope with illness?

Psychological and social factors and processes that affect how people cope with threats to health are covered in this chapter. The chapter also describes 'thinking' factors such as health beliefs and family patterns relating to health problems that may, in turn, influence our reactions to being unwell.

Chapter 4 – Managing the physical and emotional symptoms of illness

This chapter presents information on coping with the physical as well as the emotional symptoms, using mindfulness and cognitive behavioural ideas. Evidence suggests that our focus and thinking about symptoms affect the intensity with which we experience them, as well as the impact they have on our lives. In this chapter, mindfulness skills are outlined in relation to 'dropping the struggle' with chronic and persistent symptoms.

Particular attention is paid to adjusting to reduced energy levels and physical resources. This chapter will help you to pace activities over the course of a day and a week, and to conserve energy for the ones which are most important to you.

Chapter 5 – Managing anxiety in the context of illness

This chapter describes the nature of anxiety issues ranging from fear (which is a very common reaction) to the clinical anxiety which can be triggered by illness and which is more severe. We also address the uncertainty and worry which commonly present in the face of acute or chronic health conditions. The chapter provides cognitive behavioural strategies for managing and coping with anxiety and preventing its increasing in severity.

Chapter 6 – Managing depression in the context of illness

Low mood and hopelessness are common psychological reactions and responses to a diagnosis of chronic or acute illness. This chapter describes the range of experiences, from non-clinical low mood to more severe presentations of depression. As well as discussing the complexities of identifying such issues in the presence of a health condition, the chapter provides cognitive behavioural and mindfulness strategies for coping with these symptoms and also signposts where and how to obtain more specialist help in the case of more severe problems.

Chapter 7 – Managing self-esteem in the context of illness

Low self-esteem due to the physical and social changes brought about by health problems is common. These can include changes in life roles, ability to work or physical appearance, as well as social and emotional functioning. Low self-esteem can cause or worsen symptoms associated with anxiety and low mood. This chapter presents a range of cognitive and behavioural approaches to coping with low self-esteem.

Chapter 8 – Talking to friends and family

It is well established that social support has a major influence on reducing anxiety, depression and stress for people affected by health problems. This chapter looks at how you can engage your natural support system, including friends, family, voluntary agencies and the extended community, in sustaining you through your illness. It includes guidance on establishing who is the best person to talk to, and how and when to do this. We also include advice on preparing for and responding to negative or upsetting reactions from others and how to set up continuing support.

Chapter 9 – Making the most of support from your medical team

Complex medical problems will inevitably link you to a professional network of caregivers, most of whom will not have been a part of your life before you became ill. This chapter focuses on learning who the different professionals are, their relationships with you and how to manage these relationships effectively. We also provide advice on helpful sources of information and the benefits of taking control and researching your condition usefully, as well as highlighting some of the pitfalls of accessing unfiltered information on the internet.

Chapter 10 – How to support a friend, partner or family member who is unwell

This chapter is written with caregivers in mind, and includes practical ways to help support and listen to the unwell person during a complicated and at times fraught journey.

Chapter 11 – What to do if this book is not enough

We recognize that a self-help book of this type cannot cover every aspect of your situation, so in this final chapter we highlight where more specialist help may be indicated.

2

Typology of medical conditions

There are many books on how people react to and cope with a range of specific medical conditions. These books most usually reflect people's experience of living with cancer, diabetes, coronary heart disease, HIV disease, acute psychiatric problems and certain neurological conditions such as multiple sclerosis and Parkinson's disease.

It is not possible within the limits of this book to address these (or other) specific medical conditions in detail. If you need information and guidance for one of these – or any other chronic or acute disease – this is best obtained directly from the medical professionals involved in your care, or from one of the support organizations dedicated to that particular medical condition. Nor is it our intention here to discuss, or even list, all the different symptoms, reactions to medication or possible psychological responses anyone can have; instead, we want to help you understand generally how the nature or type of medical condition you are experiencing is likely to affect you. In this chapter, we aim to describe a framework for thinking about how different medical conditions affect people psychologically.

How you react psychologically to being unwell will depend on a number of different factors. These include: the nature of the condition – whether it is acute, chronic, life-threatening or a combination of any of these; whether it is treatable or curable; the extent and quality of the support you have around you; and of course the effects of the condition on your physical and mental capacities, among many others. Every health condition is different and each individual will be affected in different ways. It is true to say that no two people ever respond in the same way, even though they may be suffering from the same condition.

There are common patterns that can be observed in the responses to different medical conditions and the people affected by them. However, your reaction to a health issue is mainly determined by your personal, social and medical contexts. It is therefore important to understand more about these factors, which are likely to influence your psychological reaction to living with a serious health condition, and particularly how these are likely to influence your mood and your levels of anxiety.

> Sara heard that her best friend Yasmin was off work with flu. She had a number of brief thoughts. First, she thought that her friend would in all likelihood survive this unpleasant and unwelcome episode of ill health. Second, she thought that her friend would be off work for a short while and probably feel emotionally at a low ebb. Yasmin complained of fever and a lack of energy due to her body spending its resources on fighting the infection. Sara assumed that her friend would feel less like socializing and she did not want to see her in case she caught her infection. The good news was that Yasmin's illness, although unpleasant and an interruption to her daily life and Sara's interaction with her, wasn't life-threatening and Sara knew that Yasmin would soon be better and back to normal.

> By contrast, when Sara learned that her uncle had suffered a heart attack she wondered how bad it was. Was his condition life-threatening? Had someone telephoned the emergency services? What did he go through before receiving medical help? She pondered the circumstances: where did he suffer the heart attack? Was he alone? She considered the impact on her uncle's family and wondered how they were coping. She was really worried about whether her uncle had to have surgery or some other invasive treatment to repair any damage done by the heart attack or to prevent any future occurrence or episode. She also considered the long-term effects, both on her uncle and on her wider family.

These two seemingly different scenarios, stemming from apparently different medical conditions, can also produce very different responses in the friend concerned. How many of us have friends who have gone down with flu and have described themselves as feeling as if they are dying? By contrast, some people who suffer acute medical episodes play down their experience and suffering, seeming calm and relatively unworried, not wanting to alarm or cause anxiety to their loved ones. The above examples are given to introduce the concept of **typology of medical conditions**. Health conditions can be grouped according to particular features or characteristics. These characteristics typically reflect the nature of the **onset**, **course**, **outcome** and **degree of incapacitation** an illness or condition may bring.

Disease onset

Onset of disease refers to the length of time a disease takes to appear. For example, some conditions may develop and present gradually over time, such as with Alzheimer's disease or motor neurone disease. With these illnesses, there is more time for people and their loved ones to adjust to and prepare for specific stages or symptoms. The affected individuals also have more time to cope emotionally with and adjust to the changes brought about by their condition. By contrast, rapid, acute or sudden onset of a medical condition normally triggers significant psychological distress. An example is a stroke or heart attack – the speed and suddenness with which these conditions present is likely to cause significant emotional upheaval and distress in a far shorter period of time than with a disease of gradual onset.

Disease course

Chronic diseases can differ quite markedly in the extent to which they develop or progress. Some conditions become worse over time, entailing a deteriorating quality of life. Without medical intervention or any known and effective treatments, conditions such as Alzheimer's disease and motor neurone disease mostly worsen over time. Other conditions are constant and can remain relatively stable or even static over time. This may be due to the nature of the condition or be brought about by certain medications, many of which have to be lifelong. Examples of relatively stable medical conditions are osteoarthritis or well-managed diabetes.

There are some forms of progressive and chronic health conditions that may entail fluctuating periods of stability. The individual may enjoy predictable health and relative wellbeing for various periods, although this can be interrupted by dramatic setbacks, relapses or sudden deterioration to a lower level of functioning. Examples are some forms of cancer, multiple sclerosis or cardiac disease. This type of condition is often termed 'relapsing–remitting' because of these patterns of fluctuation between periods of stability and instability.

Disease outcome

Some chronic diseases are characterized as 'fatal' or 'non-fatal', depending on the ultimate outcome. This may seem crude or insensitive, but in a book such as this, which deals with the sensitive topic of coping with severe health problems, it is sometimes necessary to define things properly and definitely. With a fatal chronic disease, the disease may contribute to a shortening of lifespan and, almost inevitably, periods of chronic ill health, incapacity, dependency and, for some perhaps, pain. Non-fatal chronic diseases do not necessarily run a predictable course; it is possible that the person will experience times of ill health but at other times may be free of symptoms. In some cases it is possible that the underlying condition is a final contributory cause of death, while not being the direct cause. For example, somebody with chronic heart disease that is well managed and controlled may suffer a stroke or kidney disease because of his or her heart condition.

There are some diseases which currently almost inevitably entail predictable deterioration and, in all likelihood, death. Pancreatic cancer is an example of this; it is currently possible to manage some of the symptoms associated with the disease, but it is in the end incurable and, as such, requires the person and his or her loved ones to adapt to the inevitability of the processes of dying and death.

Degree of incapacitation

The specific nature of a disease may or may not have an effect on someone's ability to cope independently of medical and social support. Similar conditions may result in a much greater degree of incapacitation and dependency for some people than others, and therefore the degree to which the person draws on the resources and support of loved ones also differs widely. For example, someone with Parkinson's disease may experience significant incapacity and this may require family members to provide a high level of social, physical and financial support. An older adult, by contrast, with a form of cancer that is treatable and manageable may not need to rely on loved ones until the final stages of the disease. The actual disease is not so much the question here as the response of the person to that disease.

Note that the typology of medical conditions as it relates to the onset, course, outcome and degree of incapacitation affects not only the person but also the loved ones to whom that person turns for support. Everyone may be profoundly affected emotionally. Depression and anxiety are the most common psychological experiences reported by everyone involved, and for which they may seek help. We address the impact on family relationships more extensively in Chapter 8.

Attribution

It is generally observed that people react differently to chronic health conditions, depending on how the condition was contracted in the first place. This can sometimes help shed light on how people cope in their varying ways with different conditions. Someone who, for example, is wheelchair-bound because of a road traffic accident caused by a drink-driver may in certain ways react differently to this unwelcome situation from someone in the same situation because of a genetic disease. Someone who contracts HIV in unprotected sexual intercourse with an infected partner may experience feelings that are different from those of a haemophiliac infected in the early 1980s by a contaminated blood transfusion. This is not to introduce complex issues relating to 'blame', which are beyond the scope of this book, but more to focus on the psychological concept of **attribution**. Attribution is about how we understand things happening in the world.

The catastrophe of the 2004 Indian Ocean tsunami, for example, was an act of nature or an act of God (according to your point of view). The emotional reaction to loss in this type of catastrophic situation is different from the reaction to loss caused by poor sanitation or lack of food due to international politics, or by 'lifestyle' diseases such as liver disease linked with alcohol misuse or psychosis caused by recreational drug misuse. How and to what we attribute illness in part influences our emotional reaction, but this does not always tell the whole story.

Control

Psychological reactions to chronic disease may be affected not only by the degree of incapacitation we experience but also by the extent to which we can control or manage our condition. For example, with hypertension (high blood pressure) advice may be given to change what we eat, start exercising, lose weight and take specific medication. If these interventions are successful, then we may feel more confident about managing our condition, and we therefore become more hopeful about it. By contrast, there are some conditions where we are wholly reliant on medication and other outside interventions, and in these circumstances we may feel passive about our situation and therefore perhaps less hopeful.

An understanding of the main characteristics of your condition is important in order to determine how it may affect you psychologically.

While it may be helpful to consult specific books or turn to support organizations dealing with particular conditions, a good starting point would be to examine the four dimensions of the health problem: onset, course, outcome and degree of incapacitation, as explained earlier. It is not always necessary to have an extensive understanding of a particular medical condition in order to know how you may be affected. As we have stressed throughout this chapter, it is impossible to predict how any one individual will be affected by a particular illness. Furthermore, an understanding of how you came to be ill in the first place, and extending this understanding to your broad psychological experiences in life such as your development of resilience, your previous experience of illness and family patterns in dealing with health conditions, can all shed further light on your emotional state and condition and those of your loved ones.

Psychological support

Psychological support can help you to cope better with your physical condition. People diagnosed with serious health problems handle the challenges this presents in a variety of ways. Some find that psychological counselling is helpful to them, and to their partner, family, loved ones and friends. Taking advantage of psychological counselling and support does not mean that you have a psychological problem. Mental illness is quite different and distinct from psychological coping and adjusting to living with a specific challenge, such as a long-term health condition. Any significant personal, financial, social, emotional or other challenge in someone's life is likely to cause stress and worry, and at times there may be physical symptoms such as sleep disturbance, appetite problems, low mood and perhaps a sense of not seeing the wood for the trees. The problem becomes overwhelming, seemingly insoluble, and thinking patterns become rigid and repetitive. These are normal reactions to abnormal life events, and psychological counselling can help. Psychological counselling and therapy can also help with specific challenges that can arise as a consequence of being diagnosed with a serious health problem, such as telling your children or coping with some of the physical challenges you experience.

Four key factors are important in adjusting to chronic or acute medical problems and the psychological impact on you and the people you love:

1 good support from family and friends;
2 open communication between people about what is happening
   and what to prepare for in the future;
3 managing illness, specific symptoms, effects of treatment, stress,
   worry and uncertainty in practical and effective ways;
4 an open and supportive relationship with your doctor and other
   medical professionals.

Coping with the psychological effects of illness does not mean having
to cope on your own. Good coping means being open to the support
of family members, friends, professional caregivers and people from
voluntary organizations too.

3

What affects how we cope with illness?

Being unwell affects people in very different ways. In the last chapter we considered the ways in which different types of health issues can have a different impact on your life and the life of those around you. While some of the differences in people's responses are related to which condition they have, other factors have to be taken into account. Two people who have a very similar condition can respond very differently indeed. In this chapter we will explore some of the key factors and processes that impact on how people cope with illness.

Life cycle

Where we are in our life cycle is a key factor that influences how people and their families cope and adjust to living with being unwell. Whether the person with the condition is a newly born infant, a child, an adolescent, an adult or an older adult is likely to have a significant impact on how the individual, as well as those around him or her, responds to the illness. For example, if the grandfather of a family is diagnosed with heart failure at 87 years old, this might have a different impact on a family from a 4-year-old boy being diagnosed with a serious heart problem.

How a couple manage one of them being diagnosed with a health problem is also affected by where they are in the span of their relationship. If they have recently met, are newly wed or are a couple facing an 'empty nest' or retirement, this will also have an effect on coping.

Roles

The role that you have in your family is also relevant. Whether you are already dependent on other members of the family to some degree or are the breadwinner can play a part in how you cope with the condition. Sometimes people in particular roles feel less able to communicate their distress to those around them. For example, as a parent you may put significant energy into hiding your fears to protect your children.

Family patterns of coping

The way that people close to you, including your family, tend to cope with difficulty in general is likely to affect how you respond to health problems. In a family where people are encouraged to keep their feelings to themselves and to not show others that they are struggling, members are much less likely to share their fears and struggles with those around them. In contrast, in a family where people have always been encouraged to be open and honest about their feelings, members are more likely to open up to others.

Personality

Personality is viewed as the combination of particular enduring traits within our character that differentiate us from others. Particular personality traits might affect how we cope with a health problem. For example, if you are prone to being optimistic and extroverted, that may influence how you cope and use the support from people around you.

Previous experience of adversity

Whether you and/or your friends and family have experienced adversity before and your previous responses to it can be another factor, whether your previous experiences of adversity were health-related or not. It can be helpful to ask yourself:

• How did I cope before?
• What and who helped me to cope in that situation?

If you have not coped with an adverse situation of this scale before, it may be helpful to consider whether you know people who have. Some people find it helpful to draw from role models within their social and familial circles whose resilience they have admired during a difficult time.

- What and who was it that helped them to cope in that way?
- What did they stand for in the face of adversity that I respected?

It may then be helpful to consider in what ways you can use your own previous coping strategies, or those of other people, to help build your own resilience and coping skills and apply them to this situation.

Lifestyle factors

The way we spend our time from day to day can affect how we cope with medical problems. In general, people cope better if they remain active and engaged in their life, be it in their work, socially or physically. In Chapter 4 we look further at the relationship between lifestyle and experiences of depression and low mood.

Whether you are working, unemployed or retired will have an impact on how you cope with health difficulties, depending on the type of condition and work. Some people can continue to work alongside managing their condition and this can help them to maintain a sense of normality. Others might have to leave work because of their health and this can create a number of issues relating to identity and self-esteem, discussed further in Chapter 7. If you have to leave work because of your health, there are also very real financial issues to contend with, which can lead to further stress.

Social support

The extent to which people feel supported by those around them can significantly impact on how they cope with being unwell. Social support can come from a partner, family members, friends, neighbours, your wider community and, increasingly, online communities (e.g. online support groups for people with similar conditions).

The amount that you feel supported does not always relate to the number of people around you. The quality of the support you experience is usually more important.

Sheetal is 38 and lives with her husband and her three children. When she was diagnosed with breast cancer her immediate and extended family and her friends rallied around. All the family brought round food, did the household chores, looked after the children and drove her to her hospital appointments. From the outside it seemed as though Sheetal had a great deal of support. However, Sheetal was feeling very scared, angry and sad about her cancer diagnosis and treatment, and whenever she tried to talk to friends and family about this she was told to 'be positive'. Sheetal's friends and family said this because they did not want her to feel bad; however, it actually meant that Sheetal did not feel able to express any of her fears or feelings about what she was experiencing. As a result Sheetal felt very alone and unsupported emotionally.

The final section of the book will provide information about how to improve and make the most of the support available to you.

How we relate to health professionals

For some people, asking for help and trusting health professionals can be straightforward. However, this is not the case for everyone. Some find it very difficult to put their trust in people they have only just met. Likewise, it can feel natural to some people to challenge health professionals and ask questions, whereas others can find this very uncomfortable. How you relate to the different professionals will be influenced by your previous experiences of healthcare as well as your cultural beliefs. This can significantly impact on your experience and management of the condition and how supported you feel. For this reason we have devoted a chapter to this in the final section of this book.

Health beliefs

The way in which you make sense of your illness and what it means to you will affect how you feel about it. Throughout our lives, as we are trying to make sense of the world around us, we develop beliefs. These beliefs are shaped by our life experiences. We develop beliefs about ourselves (e.g. 'I am weak'), the world we live in (e.g. 'The world is a hostile and dangerous place'), relationships (e.g. 'Everyone I get close to leaves me'). Once these beliefs are established, they serve as a framework through which we continue to make sense of the world. You can think of them as being like a lens in a pair of glasses. You will generally make sense of your day-to-day experiences through the lens of these beliefs. For example, if you have experienced violence, hostility and unpredictability in your childhood, you may develop the belief that 'the world is a dangerous place'. This belief could mean that you feel more threatened than most other people do in a range of situations. For example, if you were lost in a new part of town and needed to ask for directions, you might feel very anxious about being lost and concerned about whether you could trust anyone enough to ask for directions. On the other hand, someone who has developed the belief that 'other people are generally good and trustworthy' is likely to experience the situation differently and may feel more comfortable about approaching a stranger and asking for help.

Your experience of a situation will depend on the situation itself as well as the beliefs you hold. Sometimes these beliefs can be helpful and sometimes they can make a difficult situation even harder.

We develop beliefs about health, just as we do about other areas of life. We know that the beliefs we develop about health can significantly influence how we make sense of and respond to being unwell. Our experiences of health and illness within our family and our community significantly influence the beliefs we develop. Whether you have had previous experience of being unwell, whether people close to you have developed health problems and how they have responded to illness, and how individuals have coped with the challenges of being unwell will all shape the ideas, assumptions and beliefs you hold about health and illness and what it means.

Tony is 55 years old. He is married with two children. After a coronary angiogram his cardiologist told him that he had coronary heart disease. Heart surgery was strongly advised to bypass the diseased area, in order to reduce the risk of heart attack. Tony experienced high levels of anxiety at the prospect of surgery, which would involve opening up the chest and operating on the heart directly. While it would be absolutely natural to be nervous about such major surgery, Tony's anxiety was affecting him very significantly. He was not able to sleep, his appetite was reduced, he avoided spending time on his own and he also avoided leaving the house. Tony could not stop worrying about the surgery and about his health. He was also delaying the date of the surgery, which was putting him at greater risk of having a heart attack and becoming more unwell. Tony felt hopeless and low in mood. He thought that there was no point in going for the surgery because he believed he would die soon. Indeed, Tony believed that he 'could die any minute' from his heart disease and that he would not survive the surgery. While doctors had reassured him that the surgery was safe and would significantly improve his health, this did not change Tony's mind.

When Tony met a psychologist and talked about his experiences of being unwell, he explained that both of his parents had died from heart problems soon after being diagnosed with cardiac conditions. He had an uncle and a brother who had also been seriously disabled by a series of strokes and had had to live in care homes for the rest of their adult lives. Tony's grandparents had also all died relatively suddenly, some of heart disease and some of cancer.

In his conversations with the psychologist it became clear that Tony's life experience had developed his health belief that 'serious illness means that your life is over'. He had learned that becoming unwell led to either early death or lifelong serious disability, and this was significantly affecting how he made sense of his current situation. When he first discussed this, Tony could not recall any examples or stories that showed him that people can recover when they become unwell, or that they can learn to live well with their condition. When Tony was thinking about his heart condition and his surgery through the lens of his health belief, it meant that he felt that his life was over, and this led him to feel terrified about dying – it was hardly surprising that he felt low in mood.

Tony's belief led him to perceive the risk of him not surviving and recovering from his surgery was close to 100 per cent, although this was not the case in reality. This meant that his levels of distress were disproportionate to the actual risk that he faced.

In addition to our past experiences, the culture in which we are embedded can significantly affect the beliefs we develop about health. All cultures have ways of explaining the causes of illness, how it should be treated and who should be involved in the treatment. These cultural health beliefs can shape our own beliefs without us being consciously aware of it. Some cultures take a fatalistic view of illness, believing that it is punishment for sins in this life or a previous one and that 'God's will' will determine the outcome. In some cultures, an elder within the family will hold the responsibility for making decisions about healthcare for others in the family. Where they exist, such cultural health beliefs are likely to have shaped both the family's and the community's response to illness.

As we have described, health beliefs are key in how individuals and their families respond to, make sense of, manage and cope with being unwell. As we saw with Tony, sometimes these health beliefs can be unrealistic and very unhelpful. In Tony's situation, his health beliefs caused him huge amounts of anxiety and also led to him putting himself at more risk. For this reason it is important to identify what your health beliefs are so that you are able to consider whether they are helpful or unhelpful. And if you decide they are unhelpful, then you can consider changing how much you pay attention and listen to these beliefs.

Here are some steps to follow to help address unhelpful health beliefs.

Identify your health beliefs

When trying to identify your health beliefs, think about the messages you were given about health and illness when you were growing up and throughout your life. Ask yourself the following questions:

- How was health and illness talked about at home?
- What experiences did you have of being unwell?
- What experiences did other people around you have of being unwell?
- How did the other people around you respond when someone else was unwell or died?
- How did your family or community make sense of these difficult events?
- Do you know people who survived or managed a serious health conditions?
- How did the people around you make sense of their survival or recovery?
- Do you have religious beliefs that influence how you think about health and illness?
- What beliefs are there within your wider culture that might shape your beliefs about health and illness?

To help you identify your health beliefs we have listed some common unhelpful health beliefs which we have come across in our work with clients:

- Illness is a sign of weakness.
- Illness is a punishment for bad behaviour in earlier life.
- Taking medication means you are an old person.
- Illness is a means of getting attention from others.
- You cannot experience happiness if you have an illness.
- No one wants to be around people with illness.
- If you pretend it is not happening, illness might go away.
- Doctors should not be trusted.
- Your illness is evidence that everything bad happens to you.
- Negative thinking makes you more unwell.

- Illness means that your life is over.
- Illness affects the way other people see you.
- Your illness defines your identity.
- You have no control over your illness.
- Medicines are society's way of controlling you.
- Illness means you are alone.
- You cannot tolerate discomfort.

Notice when your health beliefs come to mind

Once you have identified your health beliefs, it is important to start to notice when they are triggered and how they affect your thinking in everyday situations. This involves learning to 'step back' from your thoughts and notice when your health beliefs are influencing your thinking. What situations tend to trigger your belief? What are the times that you tend to think in this way? A key part of this step is to notice that your health beliefs are just beliefs; they are stories that your mind is telling you about what it means to be ill and they are not necessarily true or helpful. You may find that as soon as you start to notice that these are just beliefs and not facts, they have less of an effect on you. For Tony, when he found himself feeling very anxious, he would check in with his thinking. The moment he noticed that his 'illness means your life is over' belief was triggered, he would feel better because he would remember that this belief was just a thought and not a fact.

One way to step back and remember that this is just a thought is to preface your thinking with the sentence 'I am thinking the thought that . . .' For example, Tony would say, 'I am thinking the thought that illness means your life is over.' As soon as he did this he felt more distanced from the thought and it had a less profound effect on him.

Ask yourself, is this belief helpful?

When you have noticed your beliefs, you can ask yourself the following questions:

- Is thinking this helpful?
- Is holding on to this belief helping me to cope with this situation?
- Is it helping me to live the life I want to live, now?

For Tony the answer was definitely 'no'. Holding on to the belief meant that he was experiencing high levels of distress, which meant that he couldn't concentrate, couldn't sleep and had lost his appetite. He was irritable with his wife and children and he didn't want to leave his flat. He was also avoiding the surgery, which put him at a dangerous risk of having a heart attack and becoming considerably more unwell. He realized that by holding on to this belief he was actually putting himself at greater risk of becoming very unwell.

Deon is a 17-year-old boy who has recently been diagnosed with type-1 diabetes. His mother has managed a chronic skin condition for the last 15 years and his grandmother has managed rheumatoid arthritis for the past 10 years. Deon has the belief that 'my diabetes is a part of me but does not define who I am'. He developed this belief through observing his mother and grandmother effectively manage health conditions while still living rich and fulfilling lives. Deon has seen people around his mother and grandmother recognize their health conditions but still treat them as 'normal'. Deon finds that this health belief is helpful because it allows him to attend to and manage his diabetes when he needs to but also to focus on other parts of his identity and his life as a 17-year-old boy.

If you are unsure whether the belief is helpful or not, it may be useful to consider the pros and cons of holding on to that belief. It may be that you decide it is helpful, like Deon's, and that you do not want to challenge or change how you respond to it.

Challenge the belief

These beliefs are stories that your mind is telling you and they are often biased, particularly negative and unhelpful. It can be helpful to challenge the truthfulness of your health belief to help you to see that it is just a belief and not a fact.

When Tony was first asked by his psychologist if he knew anyone who had survived or managed an illness he had said that he didn't. Tony was later encouraged by his psychologist to think harder about this. She recommended that he speak to his wife, his friends and his colleagues about their experiences of being unwell. Tony came back to his next session with a long list of people he knew who had had major operations and health conditions and were doing well. He learned about his wife's aunt who had survived breast cancer, his friend who had survived a heart attack and another friend who had survived testicular cancer. He even found out that three years previously one of his colleagues had had the same operation as he was due to have and had recovered well. When he was looking at his situation through the lens of his health belief 'serious

ins that your life is over', he could only remember stories
ed up his belief: examples of people who had died or been
itly disabled by health problems. Tony found that doing this
rese.   and hearing all these stories about people who had recovered
well from surgery and illness helped him to challenge his health belief,
and to believe it less. He found that when he believed it less, it did not
have such a strong effect on him and he started to believe that people
could recover and manage serious health problems.

A helpful way to challenge your beliefs and thoughts is to draw up a
list of all the evidence that supports your belief and all the evidence
that doesn't support it. We recommend that you get other people
involved with this process too. If you ask around, you will often hear
of alternative experiences of health and illness and these can help to
challenge your own assumptions and beliefs. You may find that you
gather evidence that is contrary to your belief and this may help you
to believe it less and form a more helpful alternative belief. Here are
some other helpful questions to ask yourself when challenging your
belief.

- Who would disagree with this view?
- What might that person know about being ill that I don't?
- What would I say to my best friend if he or she held this belief/
  thought?
- What events suggest that this is not true?
- Is this true 100 per cent of the time?
- Am I falling into the trap of negatively skewed thinking?
- Are there any exceptions to this rule?
- What other opinions do people hold?
- Is there a more helpful or realistic way of thinking?

Tony's challenges to his health belief are shown in Table 3.1, overleaf.
Sometimes people find it difficult to challenge their health belief
and to find the evidence to help them to believe it less. If this is the
case, then you can still ask yourself whether thinking in this way is
helpful for you at this time. Is focusing on these particular thoughts
helping you to cope? If you decide that it is not helpful, then you
can continue to notice when the belief is triggered, remembering that
it is a belief and not a fact. If it is not helpful for you to think in
this way, then shift your focus on to something else in that moment.
In the chapters that follow we pay more attention to challenging

Table 3.1 Challenging Tony's health belief

Situation	Health belief and negative thoughts associated with it	Evidence against the thought/belief
Doctor telling me I need to book my surgery as soon as possibe.	I will not survive the surgery. The surgery will mean that I will be permanently disabled.	John from work said that the recovery was painful but that he felt much better after the surgery. My wife's friend had the surgery and she recovered well. The longer I put off the surgery the more risk I have of having a heart attack. My family wants me to be safe and healthy and they want me to have this surgery.

thoughts, managing thoughts that are negative but realistic, and letting unhelpful thoughts go.

In this chapter we have considered some of the factors and processes that influence how individuals and their families and friends respond to illness. The good news is that there is much you and those around you can do to improve how you respond to your health issues. The following chapters will go into greater detail on most of the topics touched upon in this chapter and will provide practical strategies to change unhelpful patterns, with a view to helping you improve how you respond to and manage your own health issues.

4

Managing the physical and emotional symptoms of illness

When diagnosed with an illness you can find yourself having to learn to cope with a range of physical symptoms, which can be difficult. A broad range of emotional experiences usually accompanies physical symptoms, and these too can present significant challenges. This chapter explores some of these experiences and looks at how they interact. We consider how unhelpful patterns and cycles can be formed, and then consider the management of physical and emotional symptoms using CBT and mindfulness skills. We also pay particular attention to the management of fatigue and explore some strategies that can be helpful with this.

Identifying unhelpful patterns

Colin had a heart attack and was diagnosed with coronary heart disease. This came as a huge shock to him, and afterwards he felt very anxious about having another heart attack. He kept getting stuck in the cycle of interactions that we looked at in Chapter 1 (see Figure 1.1, p. 6).

- *Thoughts* He would spend time worrying about having another heart attack and scanning his chest area for any new and potentially dangerous symptoms.
- *Feelings* Anxiety, fear.
- *Behaviour* He would tend to stop what he was doing and scan his body for symptoms. Occasionally he would search on the internet for information on particular sensations he was experiencing, hoping for reassurance. However, because he was focused on the worst-case scenario, he would be drawn to websites with all sorts of information suggesting these sensations were deadly. This only served to increase his anxiety.

- *Body* His breathing would become fast and shallow, his heart rate would increase and he would feel hot and start to sweat. He also felt agitated and his hands would start to shake.

Because these symptoms were similar to those of a heart attack, they increased his anxiety further. However, they were actually the result of his anxiety rather than a cardiac event. When we feel anxious our bodies go into 'fight or flight mode' and this can trigger all the bodily symptoms that Colin was noticing.

Colin was 'scanning' his body for sensations, which meant that he was much more likely to notice sensations that he might not have noticed before. This was particularly problematic at mealtimes when he would mistake feelings associated with digestion for cardiac symptoms. Colin's body was responding to his anxiety and for this reason he noticed the shortness of breath, speeding heart rate and rise in temperature and interpreted them as signs of another heart attack. As with other health conditions, the symptoms of an acute health event can overlap significantly with symptoms of anxiety. This can be very confusing and it can take some time to learn how to differentiate them. Such symptoms understandably increased Colin's worry that he was very unwell and might die, and of course this made him feel even more anxious and his symptoms intensified.

When Colin learned about his self-perpetuating cycles he realized that if he made changes to the different parts of the cycle he would feel much better. He had gone to the Accident and Emergency department several times with these symptoms, and the doctors had done tests that showed him that these symptoms were not a sign that something was wrong with his heart but were probably a result of his anxiety. As a result, he learned how to relax his body by taking slower, deeper breaths and noticed that this calmed down his body. He realized that if he started to focus on his breath in his abdomen, he stopped focusing on his experiences in his chest and felt calmer. He also learned that looking on the internet always increased his anxiety and, when he stopped doing this, his anxiety did lessen.

Throughout this book we refer to different patterns set up between our thoughts, feelings, behaviour and body. We pay particular attention to patterns in anxiety, low mood and depression, and self-esteem. In each chapter we also list helpful strategies to help you to break out of these cycles. We recommend that you try to track what is happening when you have a particularly distressing experience. If you can try to stop, step back and write down what you were thinking, doing and feeling physically, this may help you to understand the types of cycles you are getting stuck in.

Physical symptoms

When you are first diagnosed, you are likely to experience some physical symptoms. These can vary hugely in nature, intensity and persistence, depending on the nature of your illness, as is discussed in Chapter 2. Symptoms are often classified as either 'acute' or 'chronic'.

- Acute symptoms usually come and go. Examples are: palpitations, trembling and fatigue during hypoglycaemic episodes if you are diabetic, nausea as a result of chemotherapy for cancer or crushing chest pain, sweating and shortness of breath during a heart attack.
- Chronic symptoms are those that you may have to manage on a daily basis and that are unlikely to disappear. Examples of chronic symptoms are: joint pain in rheumatoid arthritis, breathlessness in chronic obstructive pulmonary disease (COPD) and heart failure, and tremors in Parkinson's disease. Additionally, some symptoms may be due to treatment or the side effects of medication.

As you can see from these examples, different symptoms call for different responses. Some are signals that something is seriously wrong and others are sensations associated with continuing processes in your body and are not harmful to you. Sudden-onset crushing chest pain means you need to go to hospital as soon as possible, which is not necessarily appropriate in, for example, a flare-up of rheumatoid arthritis pain.

When coping with symptoms it is best to become an expert on your condition. The more that you learn about your symptoms and how you should respond to them, the better equipped you will be to manage them effectively. Gather as much information as possible from your team of health professionals. They are the people who can tailor the advice to your specific situation.

When researching your condition on the internet, it is important to be selective. While there are some helpful websites with good quality information (e.g. the NHS Choices website, <www.nhs.uk/>), there are many uninformed websites containing alarmist and incorrect information that can cause unnecessary anxiety. And remember, online information is directed towards people in general and is not tailored to your specific presentation.

Symptoms diary

You may have relapsing and remitting symptoms that are chronic but flare up at different times. It is helpful to learn as much as you can about the pattern of these symptoms so that you know best how to manage them. Keep a symptoms diary, recording the pattern of your symptoms in a diary, calendar or table; search for 'symptoms diary' online for some helpful ideas. As well as noting symptoms and when they occur (day and hour), rate them out of 10 for intensity (where 10 is the most intense they have ever been and 0 indicates that they are not there). After a week or so, review your symptoms diary and look for patterns. You might be able to notice particular triggers or activities that are helpful in preventing flare-ups.

> Amir has a neuropathic pain condition. When reviewing his pain symptom diary, he noticed that his pain was always worse around times of stress. He also noticed that arguments with his wife and children tended to bring on a bad pain episode. Because it was not possible for Amir to avoid stress completely, he focused on developing the most helpful stress-management strategies so that stress had less of an impact on him physically.

Physical symptoms are usually not experienced on their own. They are generally accompanied by a package of unpleasant emotions, thoughts about the symptoms and what they mean and also patterns of behavioural responses to the symptom.

> When Amir experienced a flare-up in his pain, he would start to worry about it and would also think about how unfair it was that he experienced it (thoughts). These worried thoughts would lead to anxiety (feeling) and his thoughts about the unfairness of the pain would trigger anger (feeling). The anger and anxiety would lead Amir to tense up his muscles; his heart rate would increase and his breathing would become quicker (body). He would then stop what he was doing and sit down and try to mentally 'fight' with the pain, trying to make it go away by focusing on it (behaviour). His increased focus on the pain, as well as his physical tension and arousal from the anger and anxiety, would lead to the sensation becoming even more intense. This would then lead to more worry and thoughts of unfairness, and the cycle would be repeated and intensified.
>
> Over time Amir found that his episodes of pain were becoming more and more problematic. They were preventing him doing the activities that were important to him and he was also experiencing high levels

of distress. He developed a set of mindfulness skills that helped him to respond differently to his pain so that he did not add any further suffering to his experience. (We will consider mindfulness skills later in this chapter.)

Emotional symptoms

As discussed, physical conditions do not just bring physical symptoms. They tend also to trigger strong emotional reactions, and these vary hugely from person to person. It is common for people to report feeling:

- shock and confusion;
- feelings of being overwhelmed;
- low feelings and hopelessness;
- anger;
- loss;
- despair;
- helplessness;
- jealousy;
- guilt;
- fear (about the future, ill health, death, dying, relationships, treatments, procedures, sexuality);
- isolation and loneliness.

And many more . . .

All these experiences are natural responses and, while they are unpleasant, they are not necessarily problematic. When something happens that has the potential to jeopardize something we care about, our response is likely to be one of strong emotions. While emotions can feel very uncomfortable and intense, it is important to remember that they are perfectly natural and that we are designed to be able to tolerate them. In fact, it is often our responses to emotions rather than the emotions themselves that are the problem.

Avoidance

Usually if we don't like something we try to avoid it, and may spend a huge amount of time and energy trying not to feel a particular emotion. In Chapter 3 we talked about Tony, who was scared about having cardiac surgery. As he really disliked feeling anxious, he tried to avoid his anxiety. This meant that he avoided thinking about the forthcoming operation or his health condition. He avoided seeing friends in case they asked him about his health, and would not leave his small flat. He would sit in the bedroom to avoid speaking to his family, watching television all day to distract himself. He avoided moving around physically so as not to increase his heart rate (because that would make him worry about his health) but indulged in drinking beer and eating his favourite comfort foods to try to relax. None of this worked in the long run. In fact, his anxiety was getting worse and worse. In addition he was feeling disconnected, lonely and increasingly bored and low in mood.

Rumination

Rumination happens if you get caught up in a particular feeling, and brood repetitively on the thoughts connected with that feeling. When Amir experienced pain, he would stop what he was doing and focus on the pain and the anger and anxiety that accompanyied it. He would get caught up in mental battles against his pain and his emotions and would ruminate on how unfair it was that he had this pain. He would get 'locked in' to these experiences for long periods of time, following his thoughts round and round. During this time his levels of distress would escalate and escalate.

Mindfulness skills can help people improve their response to difficult emotions by learning how to allow and observe difficult feelings and let them go rather than avoiding or getting caught up in them.

Mindfulness

Mindfulness skills have been shown to be effective in helping people manage physical and emotional symptoms in the context of illness and physical conditions.

Mindfulness-based therapies differentiate between primary and secondary suffering. Primary suffering refers to the symptoms themselves: the physical sensations associated with a particular health issue. However, often we don't just experience the primary symptoms in isolation. They are usually accompanied by other experiences. For example, if we experience pain we will experience the physical sensations of pain (primary suffering) and this is largely unavoidable. We will also experience thoughts about the pain (e.g. 'I wish this pain would go away', 'I can't handle it', 'It's not fair'). It is likely that there will also be emotions related to the pain (e.g. anger, anxiety, despair). The thoughts and feelings about the pain are called secondary suffering, and this can serve to make the experience of the symptoms (primary suffering) harder and more distressing. We saw this clearly in the example of Amir and his pain.

Mindfulness-based therapies provide a framework in which you can change the way you relate to the symptoms themselves, so that you do not add a secondary layer of suffering. Mindfulness suggests that we drop the struggle with symptoms (primary suffering) in order to keep the overall experience of suffering to a minimum. It is suggested that it is the struggle with the symptoms that makes them worse, so that they take up more of our energy and time. Mindfulness-based therapies suggest that we should learn to be accepting of symptoms (if it is established that they are chronic and safe) rather than struggling and fighting with them. Mindfulness practice and meditation suggest techniques to help manage symptoms more objectively and positively.

It is beyond the scope of this book to teach mindfulness in detail but here is an introductory exercise (see 'Further reading' on pages 109–10 if you want to explore mindfulness further).

Mindfulness-based breathing exercise

The essence of mindfulness is to observe the unfolding present moment non-judgementally. In a mindfulness exercise you watch the content of your experiences, such as feelings, sensations and even the wandering of the mind. At the same time you notice that these events are transient and always changing.

This exercise focuses your attention on the breath. It is designed to help you start to notice your experiences rather than judging them as 'good' or 'bad'. In this exercise you are encouraged simply to notice your experiences rather than react to them.

First, get into a comfortable position, lying on your back or sitting in a chair or on the floor. If sitting, make sure that your back is straight and your shoulders are relaxed. At first you will need to read the instructions but when you are more familiar with the exercise you can try closing your eyes, if that feels comfortable.

Now bring your attention to your body and notice the sensations you can feel within it. Are there any physical sensations that particularly grab your attention? If so, notice these and observe them with curiosity. Now notice other sensations. What sensations are there at the points in which your body is in contact with something? Can you feel contact from the floor or the chair, or from your clothing?

Now bring your attention to your lower abdomen and see if you can observe the movement of the lower abdomen in response to your breath. Can you feel it rise and expand on the in-breath and fall away on the out-breath?

Notice what other sensations are associated with your breathing.

Whenever you notice that your mind has wandered, which it will tend to do, notice what it was that drew your attention away and gently escort your attention back to the breath and the sensations of your breathing.

Focus on your breathing and follow each breath for its full duration. Notice what you can observe.

You are not trying to change or control your breath, you are simply observing it.

Time and time again your mind will wander. This is perfectly natural and there is no need to tell yourself off for it. Every time that you notice this, just gently bring your attention back to the breath.

As you are sitting still, you may notice that intense sensations might start to nag at you. This is fine. Instead of trying to ignore these sensations or trying to block them out, notice what happens if you allow them to remain in your awareness as you continue to observe your breath. When you start to notice that you are struggling with the sensation, try to replace the struggling with watching the sensation instead.

See what happens if you remain completely present to this moment without judging it, letting your thoughts come and go like cars passing on the road outside.

Continue to observe the breath. Bring the breath to the foreground of your attention, with your other experiences in the background. Allow your physical sensations and your thoughts and emotions to be there in the background and gently rest your attention on your breathing.

You may notice emotions. This is fine too. See what happens if you simply allow these emotions to be there. Observe them. See what happens when you don't struggle with the emotions and allow them to remain in your awareness while you focus on the sensations of your breathing.

Continue observing the breath, this breath coming in and this breath going out. And each time your mind wanders, bring it gently back to the next in-breath.

Now slowly come out of the exercise, open your eyes and look at the room around you. Take your time to come out of the exercise before you return to what you were doing beforehand.

How was that? Did you notice anything interesting? Did you notice what happens when you step back and observe your experiences rather than getting caught up in them?

Mindfulness is a skill that needs to be practised. It is unlikely that you will notice significant shifts after one practice. However, if you dedicate a small amount of time – say, ten minutes – each day to practising mindfulness, you may notice the following benefits:

- You become more aware of the present moment.
- There is a reduction in the amount of secondary suffering you experience alongside your symptoms.
- You learn to create distance between yourself and overwhelming symptoms by 'stepping back' from them.
- You become more able to focus your attention on what is most important to you and on what you need to do to make your life work, by allowing your symptoms and difficult internal experiences to be there in the 'background' of your attention.
- You become more engaged with others.
- There is a reduction in the overall impact of the symptoms on your life.
- You become more aware of unhelpful patterns of thinking, feeling, behaviour and body sensations.
- You become more able to observe and let go of unhelpful thoughts.

Allowing his physical and emotional symptoms just to *be* was different and difficult for Amir at first. However, he found that as he practised the exercises and learned to let go of the struggle with his symptoms, they felt different. He noticed that when he 'observed' his pain sensations and feelings, it created some distance between them and him. He found that they were less intense and distressing and more manageable. Amir noticed that his symptoms did not stay the same but changed and transformed over the course of his mindfulness practice. He found that the stories that his mind had been telling him about his pain sensations (e.g. 'I can't tolerate this') were not true. Amir found that in the mindfulness practice, as he learned to acknowledge the pain sensations and allow them to be 'in the background' of his attention, he could focus better on his breath. He then tried to apply this to his everyday life. With time he found that if difficult and uncomfortable feelings or pain came along when he was doing something that was important to him (e.g. playing with his 6-year-old daughter), he could acknowledge them, allow them to be in the background and focus his attention back on his daughter and what they were doing in the present moment. This didn't mean that the sensations disappeared, but it did mean that his attention was freed up to focus on what mattered most to him in that moment.

What shall I do if I want to learn more about mindfulness?

Mindfulness is usually taught in a group format. To find a group near you, search at <http://bemindful.co.uk/learn/find-a-course/>.

For resources about mindfulness courses specifically designed for people who are unwell, see <www.breathworks-mindfulness.org.uk/>. There are also resources that you can use on your own to learn mindfulness skills; see <www.headspace.com/> and the books listed in the mindfulness section of 'Further reading' on pages 109–10.

Fatigue

Fatigue is a very common symptom associated with illness and physical conditions. This can be because of the underlying condition itself or as a result of medication. In addition, managing a condition can be exhausting, so it is helpful to think about managing your fatigue too. There are two main points to think about: pacing and prioritizing.

Mia has a diagnosis of chronic fatigue syndrome. She has particular days where she feels as though she has energy and others when she has none at all. On a good day she used to rush around and try to get everything done before the tiredness came back – and it always did. Usually the next day she would be so incapacitated by her fatigue that she had to stay in bed for half the day and could not get anything done.

When she used a symptoms diary, Mia noticed that she would always have a 'bad day' with the tiredness following a 'good' and really busy day. From this she was able to see that her bursts of energy and activity were exhausting her for the following day – a case of 'boom and bust'. As a result, she started to pace her activity levels across the week and noticed that her fatigue tended to be more manageable, with less debilitating episodes.

Pacing

It is common for people to have a surge of activity when they are feeling well and have more energy. It is understandable that when you feel well you want to make the most of it and be as productive as possible, but this can mean that your symptoms are quite disabling when they flare up again. It is important to pace your activities and to make sure that you stop your activities *before* you are exhausted. In order to manage this, you will need to get to know your pattern of fatigue. Ask yourself:

- What are the warning signs that you are starting to get tired?
- What are the signs and signals that come before you feel exhausted?
- How can you respond to these when you notice them?
- What tends to trigger them? What helps?
- What plan should you have in place when you start to feel tired?
- How much activity is 'enough' before you should stop to prevent further exhaustion the next day?

You can then plan accordingly, and consider how to spread your activity over the day.

Prioritizing

When you have symptoms that mean it is difficult for you to do everything that you used to, it is important to prioritize, listing tasks and goals in order of importance and thinking realistically about which ones to achieve first.

- What exactly do I want or need to get done today?
- If I could only do two things today, what would they be?
- What are the things that, if I did them, would mean the most to me?
- What are the tasks or activities that I could ask someone to help me with?
- If I were to look back at today and be really pleased with myself, what would be my key achievement?
- How can I still live in line with what is important to me, even if I can't do everything I want to do?

It can be helpful to think about your values. This does not relate to moral values but, more broadly, to things that are important to you.

Simply put, values are what you want your life to stand for. Values are something that you can do on a continuing basis, such as being a supportive friend, maintaining health and fitness, being honest and loving, and so on. If it is not something you can 'do', then it is not a value. So 'happiness' is not a value. Being 'cured' is not a value as it is not something *you* can *do*. Usually, the more we live in line with our values, the more fulfilled we feel. Write down what kind of values you have and then think about the small things you could do to live more in line with them.

5

Managing anxiety
in the context of illness

This chapter describes the nature of anxiety issues, ranging from natural fear responses in the context of illness to more serious and clinical anxiety problems that can be triggered by being unwell. We describe the difficulty in identifying such issues in the context of medical problems because of the blurred lines between physical and emotional experience. Another common difficulty with health conditions is managing the worry that naturally comes when we do not know what is going to happen. This chapter provides cognitive behavioural strategies for dealing with uncertainty, anxiety and worry. These strategies will help you to identify and challenge anxious thoughts. It also applies the concept of mindfulness, and includes relaxation strategies to manage the impact of anxiety on the body.

It is hardly surprising that a diagnosis of illness is clouded with fear and dread. Being unwell may force us to confront some difficult questions, many of which we may not be able to answer. What impact will illness have on our life? How will we balance the demands of our condition with those of being a parent, or a partner? Will our work suffer? Do we fully understand what we are being told? Will we die from this disease? The uncertainty surrounding such questions can be stressful, and the answers to some of them may be daunting and frightening. However, the facts about our condition – even if they are unpleasant and frightening in themselves – will at least be a firm foundation for coping. Reliable information is very important. Much of what we hear about health problems may reflect what is at one extreme end of experience. It is natural to catastrophize, or think about all the worst possible outcomes. However, remember that being unwell is common. You are not alone – millions of people worldwide are dealing with this.

At his follow-up examination, Brian was told that his blood pressure, far from reducing as he had hoped, had actually increased and he would need further treatment. Fortunately, there were many options available. The visit to his doctor brought back many of the emotions that Brian felt when he was first diagnosed with high blood pressure. He initially felt afraid and became increasingly angry with himself for having consumed too much salt, alcohol and coffee. He became increasingly anxious about the prospect of enduring another waiting period to see if the next course of medication would take effect.

Brian wanted to appear strong and calm, feeling he had put his family and himself through enough grief the first time around because of all his dietary requirements. For the next couple of weeks he continued to suppress his fears and worries, becoming increasingly overwhelmed. It was his wife, Susan, who finally persuaded him to talk about his emotions. With her help, Brian was able to reflect on his feelings and confront his experience of anxiety and despair. He learned to look at the positive aspects of his health, such as the fact that high blood pressure is treatable. Brian was otherwise in good health and he gradually learned to overcome his fear of further health problems.

Anxiety

Anxiety is often associated with uncertainty. People may often experience anxiety:

- at the time of their diagnosis;
- when they are presenting for further investigations;
- while waiting to hear about test results;
- after receiving treatment.

Anxiety is a natural and expected response to something unknown. Indeed, it is unusual for people not to experience some degree of hesitancy, concern or worry in such circumstances. However, just as prolonged and severe sadness may be indicative of an underlying depression, so prolonged and severe anxiety may indicate a problem adjusting to the uncertainty around your illness. Severe anxieties can manifest as phobias, e.g. claustrophobia or an extreme anxiety associated with needles. These fears may interfere with assessment or treatment regimens such as CAT or MRI scans or during routine blood tests or an admission to hospital. A psychologist or counsellor can help you to learn to manage these and related symptoms of anxiety. For anxiety disorders, there are also targeted psychological and drug treatments that can be very effective.

An underlying fear about your health may always be there. If you are having difficulties coping with your treatment or if your disease is not responding to treatment, you may be afraid of what the future holds. If your condition is serious, alongside the other emotions associated with chronic or acute illness you may be confronted with the fear of not recovering, or of dying. Whatever the nature of your fears, they are normal and ones that your doctors and nurses have helped people with before, even if this is the first time that you have experienced such intense worries that you cannot resolve on your own.

Fear

Fear is a natural response to an unwelcome and potentially life-threatening event and should be accepted as such. It is not easy to challenge or confront what we are afraid of, but the goal is not to let fear dominate our life. If we let it dominate, it can have a negative impact on our quality of life, our relationships and our wellbeing.

There are constructive ways to tackle fear. These include seeking information, restructuring negative thoughts and emotions, solving problems and not avoiding exposure to certain situations. A starting point is to list the things we fear and then to talk about them to people we trust. There is a practical response to nearly everything we fear. If you feel overwhelmed by your fears or are having difficulty responding to them in a way that improves your coping, then it may be appropriate to consult a psychologist or counsellor.

Symptoms of anxiety

Anxiety is an experience that can affect people in different ways, although there are common themes and symptoms that many people share. It tends to impact on our thoughts, feelings, behaviour and physiology. Below is a list of some of the symptoms that people experience if they are feeling anxious:

- worry;
- feelings of fear and even panic;
- heightened alertness and vigilance;
- physical agitation, finding it hard to sit still;
- breathing rapidly and shallowly;
- increase in heart rate;

- avoidance of situations that trigger anxiety;
- difficulty sleeping;
- decrease or increase in weight.

In the previous chapter we described the cognitive behavioural cycle that shows how all these factors interact and tend to maintain unhelpful patterns. This is certainly true of our experiences of anxiety. The main factors that tend to keep the anxiety going are:

- avoidance;
- vigilance and focus on health and fears;
- worry and other unhelpful thinking patterns;
- heightened physiological arousal.

This chapter will offer ideas and strategies to help address all these maintenance factors in order to help you to reduce your experience of anxiety.

Reducing avoidance

Avoidance is a perfectly normal way of coping with fear. You may avoid people because of anxieties associated with having to disclose your condition to them. Avoidance can prevent you from doing things that you are capable of doing – things which could improve your quality of life. A person undergoing chemotherapy, for example, may avoid leaving the house for fear of how other people will respond to hair loss.

Avoidance due to fear is often recognized in relation to people experiencing pain. They may worry excessively about situations that could make their pain worse. While avoidance is appropriate on some occasions, such as when the pain is intense, paradoxically it can be unhelpful in others. In the long run, pain intensity may even increase if muscles become stiff or weak from lack of exercise due to avoidance. In general, avoidance tends to make people more fearful and less confident and therefore less able to manage their fears.

As we saw in the example of Tony in Chapter 3, the more he avoided thinking about his surgery, leaving the house or seeing anyone, the more anxious he became. Avoidance very often leads to an overall increase in anxiety and can mean that your illness takes over your life more than it needs to. Tony found that gathering information, speaking to friends and hearing about their own and their families' experiences of surgery and recovery helped him to feel more informed and to challenge his unhelpful beliefs. In addition, he found that when he was more active and went out of the house, he was more distracted from his worry. If you recognize that you are using avoidance, it is helpful to consider addressing your fears, but only step by step. There is more on increasing your overall levels of activity in Chapter 6, 'Managing depression in the context of illness'.

Addressing over-vigilance

Tom, a 50-year-old financial consultant, was treated for skin cancer six months ago. The doctors had caught the cancer at an early stage and the prognosis looked very positive. Tom's doctor recommended that he avoid the sun as much as possible and that he use a high-factor sunscreen during the summer. However, Tom was concerned that he would develop skin cancer again. He worried that the years he had spent surfing in South Africa as a kid had taken their toll on his skin. The worry was worse in the evenings when his mind was not distracted by work. Tom would often undress several times to check his moles in the mirror to see if they had changed colour, shape or size. He visited his GP at least once a week to ask if she could check his moles. This was in addition to regular meetings with his dermatologist. During one of his visits to the GP, Tom told the doctor that he wanted to remove all moles from his body to eliminate any risk of future skin cancer. The GP very gently explained to Tom that she had checked all his moles for several months and there was no evidence of current abnormality to any of them. She referred him to see a therapist who could help him manage his worry and fear of developing skin cancer again.

Having developed skin cancer, Tom was concerned that some of his other moles might eventually become cancerous if he did not check them on a regular basis. This is understandable. But when does being vigilant become over-vigilant and a source of excessive worry that can intensify the sense of bodily symptoms and cause a person intense feelings of stress and anxiety? This is not an easy question to answer, as there may sometimes be a fine line between being aware of illness and anticipating further health complications. Health anxiety is a form of anxiety where people are especially afraid of developing serious illness. They may therefore frequently check for physical abnormalities or visit their GP once a week or so. If you have a health condition and have become very vigilant towards your health, we advise you to discuss your concerns with your doctor.

Addressing your worry and other unhelpful thinking patterns

Worry is a form of mental problem-solving about potential negative events in the future. Often it can be helpful, because it can lead to active problem-solving and preparation for events. However, all too often we worry about things that we cannot do anything about, and the worry can become uncontrollable and get in the way of positive thinking and action. We can also catastrophize, which is when we only think of all the worst possible case scenarios.

How can you identify whether you are worrying too much? One way may be to reflect on your thinking to see if you are catastrophizing by assuming the worst. For instance, suppose you need to take sick leave from work during your treatment and are feeling anxious about telling your boss. You may feel convinced that you will lose your job despite your excellent attendance record. Is this really the case? In this and other scenarios, questions such as the following may help to challenge inaccurate thinking:

- Why do I feel anxious about taking sick leave from work? (Perhaps because I feel as if I am letting my boss or colleagues down; because my boss may have to find temporary cover for me; because, in the current economic climate, jobs may be under threat.)
- What facts might I be forgetting or ignoring? (My boss has been supportive when other colleagues have taken sick leave in the past; I have a positive attendance record at work; the oncologist has advised that I need to take time off from work to recover from my treatment and has given me a letter to this effect.)
- What is *not* true about the process of my taking sick leave from work? (That it will affect progress or promotion at work; that I may lose my job because of this; that I will personally offend my boss or my colleagues.)
- What's the worst thing that can happen? (My work will be put on hold for a couple of months; my boss won't be able to find temporary cover for me; I will feel guilty and uncomfortable.)
- How could I best handle the anxiety associated with requesting sick leave from work?

It may be helpful to list and then go over each of your current worries, one by one. Some of these may be about coping with your illness, while others may be related to your finances, family, work, living arrangements or leisure activities. It is also important to check whether any of your health beliefs have been triggered. As we discussed in Chapter 3, some people hold unhelpful health beliefs that can lead them to feel excessively anxious. When you come across an unhelpful health belief or anxiety-provoking thought, encourage more realistic thoughts by asking yourself the questions outlined in the challenging beliefs exercise in Chapter 3.

Try to address each of your anxious thoughts in turn. You may find it hard at first to generate alternatives to unhelpful thoughts because you may be so used to your negative automatic ones, but be encouraged that at least you are trying to come up with alternative ways to think about your situation and challenges.

Keeping a list of your common negative thoughts may help. You can then refer to the list in situations that make you feel upset or anxious, and may be more likely to recognize that your unhelpful thoughts have been triggered.

Letting go of worries – mindfulness practice

In some instances, challenging our thoughts will not be helpful because we may find that our fears are actually realistic. However, just because they might be realistic, it does not meant that it is helpful to continue to ruminate and focus on these worries if there is nothing we can do about them. In this instance, using mindfulness skills to let go of worry can be helpful.

Often, internal dialogue can be anxiety provoking. We tend to fast-forward into the future with worrying thoughts, delving around in uncertainty and trying to find answers that are not necessarily there. We are also prone to rewinding the past, ruminating over situations and events that we feel we could have handled better or that should have been avoidable. This type of negative thinking can be detrimental and contribute to our feelings of anxiety.

When we continually focus our attention on past and future, we run the risk of missing life in the present. As discussed in the previous chapter, mindfulness can enable us to take an observant position and to 'let go' of our worry. Here are some mindfulness techniques for managing difficult thoughts.

1 When the unhelpful patterns of thoughts come, it is important to step back and to notice that they are there.

2　Then you can ask yourself: is focusing on these thoughts helpful to me right now?

3　If the answer is no, try to let go of these thoughts using mindfulness skills by trying any of the following:

(a)　Letting the thoughts go on in the background and shifting your attention to focus on something else. Some people find it helpful to visualize their thoughts as talk on a radio station. You can imagine that rather than listening to everything on the radio, you turn down the volume and let it go on in the background. This means that you can let your thoughts continue without paying attention to them, leaving you free to focus on something else that is more helpful.

- You can focus on another activity.
- You can engage further in your surroundings and notice them. Try noticing five things that you can hear around you, five things that you can see around you and five sensations that you can feel.
- You can focus your attention on your breath, observing the breath with open curiosity as it comes in and out of your lungs

(b)　You can use imagery to help you let go of the thoughts.

- Imagine a gently flowing stream. Imagine placing your thoughts on to the stream of water and watch them float away. The thoughts may come back again. If they do, that's fine; just repeat the exercise again.
- Imagine that your difficult thoughts and feelings are like clouds in the sky. Like bad weather, your thoughts and feelings will pass. You can imagine them passing with time, and in the meantime you can focus back on the present moment.

Learn how to relax

As described in the previous chapter, when we feel anxious, it has a very real impact on our physical functioning. It increases our physiological arousal. You may notice shortened and more shallow breaths, increased heart rate, muscle tension, increase in temperature and sweating, feeling shaky. Learning relaxation skills helps you to manage the physical symptoms caused by anxiety concerning illness. It can also help to reduce pain sensations by relaxing the muscles and releasing tension. These skills will help you gain a sense of control over your unpleasant sensations and thoughts, and enable you to feel more confident emotionally. Becoming proficient in relaxation techniques will also show you that you *can* cope.

Learning how better to manage the physical symptoms of anxiety is a skill that needs to be practised frequently before you can expect to gain mastery and obtain lasting benefits. It is just like learning to drive: you need to keep practising until you are able to coordinate the many skills required to operate the car without consciously thinking about them. It can be a challenge at first, especially when trying to apply relaxation skills in a difficult situation. It is therefore important to start by practising in settings where you feel comfortable and less anxious.

Breathe slowly to restore calm

Using a simple breathing technique can help you learn to relax. The technique basically involves taking gentle breaths that fill your lungs completely, and then exhaling slowly and fully. Relaxation breathing counteracts the anxiety response and so will reduce the physical symptoms associated with anxiety. It releases tension in your body and relaxes you and, once you have managed to calm your body, it is impossible to feel strained or anxious.

1 Ensure you are sitting comfortably.
2 Slow down the rate of your breathing by breathing in deeply for three seconds, preferably through your nose. Hold for two seconds and then breathe out for four seconds through your nose or mouth.
3 Try to use your abdomen to breathe rather than just your upper chest. You can check this by placing a hand on your stomach and seeing whether you can feel it move.
4 Repeat this breathing over and over for a few minutes.

You may find it a challenge to practise controlled breathing at first, feeling as if you are not getting enough air or that the pace of your breathing seems unnaturally slow. This is a normal reaction when you practise a new routine. As your skill improves and you learn to relax quickly, you will find it easier to switch to correct breathing whenever you feel stressed.

You may want to progress to practising your breathing technique in more distracting situations and with your eyes open, such as while caught in a traffic jam or waiting outside the school gates to collect the children. The technique is simple and can be used at any stage of a stressful experience to reduce illness-induced anxiety and worry. It is easy to apply and will help to reduce tension, anxiety and pain sensations.

Releasing physical tension

When we experience anxiety we often unconsciously hold on to tension in our muscles. This can lead to further pain and discomfort and can also maintain anxiety. In a progressive muscle relaxation you tense up particular muscles and then relax them systematically. This can be very helpful as a stress management exercise.

Before starting this exercise

Only do this exercise within the limits of comfort for you. If you are concerned about it affecting your health condition, then speak to your doctor before you do this.

Try to minimize distraction to all your senses in your surroundings (e.g. turn off the TV or radio, use soft lighting).

Start by slowing down your breathing, using the calming breathing exercise above, and give yourself permission to relax.

The relaxation sequence runs through a number of muscle groups. For each muscle group, tense the muscles so that you can feel tension, but not so much that you feel pain. Keep the muscle tensed for about five seconds before you relax it. When you relax the muscle groups keep them relaxed for roughly ten seconds. Some people find it helpful to calmly say a word like 'relax' or 'calm' while they do this.

Relaxation sequence

1 Feet: curl your toes downwards.
2 Lower legs: pull your toes up towards you.
3 Upper legs: tighten your leg muscles.
4 Hips and buttocks: squeeze your buttock muscles.
5 Abdomen: tighten your abdomen muscles.
6 Shoulders: bring your shoulders up towards your ears.
7 Shoulder blades and back: push your shoulder blades back so that your chest is pushed forward.
8 Arms: hold your hands in fists and squeeze tension in your lower and upper arms.

9 Neck: facing forward, tip your head back as though you are looking up to the ceiling (take care when you tense these muscles).
10 Mouth and jaw: open your mouth as wide as you can.
11 Eyes and cheeks: squeeze your eyes shut tight.
12 Forehead: raise your eyebrows as high as they will go.

Once you have learned the skill of relaxing your muscles, your mind and body will automatically feel calmer. It is almost impossible for the mind to be anxious when the body is relaxed.

Illness-induced anxiety and worry may vary for different people. No two people are likely to react to their illness in the exact same way. People may not have the same reactions to physical illness; each of us has our own independent worry and each of us behaves differently when experiencing ill health. Some people may find that mindfulness works best for them, whereas others may prefer to challenge their anxious thoughts. It is important to find a technique that works for you. This is best done by practising the technique regularly before you use it in a stressful situation, so that you get used to doing it and gain confidence in its benefits.

Yoga

Yoga consists of a series of postures or asanas which aim to relax and strengthen both body and mind. There are a number of different yoga practices, including Hatha, Ashtanga, Bikram, Anusara, Vinyasa and Kundalini. The different types of yoga all include a concentration on posture, but each also has its own particular emphasis or difference, such as pace, intensity, use of breathing, level of physical demand or the importance placed on physical alignment and the use of chanting. The yoga postures target areas of the human anatomy such as nerves, glands and organs to stimulate enhanced functioning.

The idea of placing the body into postures is based on knowledge of the working of the anatomy and the physiology of the human body. Rather as mindfulness practice emphasizes a focus on the here and now, yoga also requires a significant amount of concentration for working the body into the postures and holding them. This means that the focus becomes the here and now, and so distracts from the ruminations and worrying thoughts that may drive feelings of fear and anger about having developed illness. The breathing techniques involved in yoga practice direct the mind to the inhaling and exhaling of breath, which can help to exclude intrusive thoughts or minimize their domination of the mind space, thus providing deeper relaxation and greater release from negative emotional states.

Choosing the yoga practice that works best for you is important. It may be that you want to just focus on gentle breathing exercises or very light stretches. Take care not to force your body or exceed your physical abilities at any time. This is an individual practice that can easily be tailored to suit the unique nature of each person.

6

Managing depression
in the context of illness

Given the psychological, social and physical challenges that are present when someone experiences the onset of illness, it is relatively common to feel low in mood and, at times, depressed. Being depressed in mood affects your behaviour in such ways that it can lead to further deterioration in your health. For this reason it is important to prioritize improving the way you feel. It is usually possible to make positive changes to your mood and for this to have a significant impact on your wellbeing. This chapter will describe the experiences of depression in the context of physical illness and the complexities associated with this. We will explore some of the unhelpful patterns that keep depression going and provide strategies to help you to break these patterns.

What is depression?

Depression is an often-used term that can have different meanings for different people. In this book we refer to depression as a cluster of symptoms that can affect our thinking, mood, motivation, concentration and sleep. It can also affect how we feel physically. It is natural for people to experience these patterns at difficult times in their lives, such as when facing illness.

There is a wide range of experiences of low mood and depression. Sometimes we can feel low in mood, experience negative thoughts and feel less motivated and interested in things than usual. These experiences can be unpleasant but tend to pass with time and are dispersed with periods when we feel all right. However, sometimes these symptoms can feel very intense, can persist for a longer period of time and can significantly impair ability to function in the different areas of life (e.g. work life, social life, relationships, etc.).

Some of the most commonly identified symptoms associated with experiences of depression are:

- low mood
- diminished motivation
- low interest in things previously of interest
- diminished pleasure in activities
- difficulty concentrating
- weight loss or weight gain
- sleeping problems
- feeling worthless and guilty
- lethargy and fatigue
- negative thinking
- reduction in activity
- withdrawing from social interactions
- more thoughts about death and suicide.

As you might have noticed, many of the symptoms on this list overlap with symptoms of some physical illnesses. As a part of their illness it is common for people to feel more fatigue and therefore experience a reduction in motivation and activity, for their sleep to be affected and for their weight to change, quite apart from any experience of low mood and depression. This means that there are often difficulties in identifying depression and low mood in the context of physical illness. On the one hand, people can have an underlying physical condition that their doctors initially misidentify as depression. On the other hand, some people who feel very low in mood have their symptoms of depression dismissed because their presentation is assumed to be part of their underlying illness.

Mohammed is 72 years old and has a diagnosis of congestive heart failure. Because the heart does not pump blood around the body as effectively, one of the most problematic symptoms in this condition is fatigue. Since his diagnosis of heart failure Mohammed had been feeling very low. He had stopped meeting friends and going to the mosque and spent more and more time in his bedroom, away from his family. Mohammed's wife was very concerned about the change in her husband and spoke to the specialist nurse about him. The nurse told her that this was very normal for people with his heart condition. She explained that because he was very tired his motivation would be lower. However, as time went on Mohammed spoke to his wife about how he was feeling. He said that as well as feeling tired he also felt very depressed. Mohammed felt ashamed about his heart failure, what it meant for his role in their household and his dependence on others. He had thoughts that he was worthless and a burden to his family now that he was unwell and was separating himself from them because of this.

When Mohammed and his medical team realized that he was feeling so low in mood, they were able to support him in making changes to improve it.

Some people experience depression as a result of side effects of treatment, for example some forms of chemotherapy and certain medications, such as Roaccutane, used to treat acne. Some types of steroids can also make people feel agitated and restless, which can affect sleeping patterns.

How to break the cycle of depression

When considering how to change a pattern, it is important to look at the factors that may be maintaining it. Common maintenance factors for depression are:

- *Reduced activity* It is common for people who feel depressed to do less and less and to withdraw from activities that usually bring relief or pleasure. Of course, the less you do what you enjoy, the worse you tend to feel and the more likely you are to get caught up in unhelpful thinking patterns.
- *Negative thinking and rumination* Low mood affects the way that we think about our lives, our future and ourselves. It leads to negatively biased thinking, where you notice only the negative and overlook the positive. Rumination is when you get stuck in repetitive thoughts, and if these are all negative then this process will make you feel very low indeed. Rumination is more likely if you spend a lot of time on your own and are relatively inactive.
- *Giving up hope* When you feel tired and low in mood your motivation will be low. This can lead to negative interpretations of whether it is worth addressing something. Rather than attempting to solve problems, you may think, 'What is the point?' This can lead to reduced attempts to manage problems, leading in turn to further hopelessness and even lower mood.

In contrast to the three factors that tend to maintain low mood, here are three techniques to help break the cycle of low mood.

1 Increasing activity levels

What we do and how we spend our time has a direct and strong effect on our mood. By structuring your time and increasing your activity levels you can significantly improve your mood.

Structure and routine

Because motivation can be very low in times of poor health, people abandon their basic routine. In addition, ill health may mean that they are working less or not at all, so that their previous routine has changed anyway. Straightforward tasks and chores can feel challenging when you are feeling low, particularly if you are spending more time at home. However, it is important to maintain your basic self-care. People are often surprised at the difference it can make to get out of bed, wash, get dressed and eat properly in the morning.

> Len had worked for 40 years as a bus driver. Two months after he retired he had a triple heart bypass. After his surgery he felt very low in mood. He had always got up early in the morning and had a shower and a shave and got dressed quickly, as he had to be out of the house very early. Now that he did not go to work and was still recovering from surgery, Len got out of bed later and later, going down to breakfast in pyjamas rather than getting dressed. He had constant negative thoughts about himself, his health and his life, and felt unmotivated to do anything with his day. He would usually then sit on the sofa to watch daytime TV, something he did not enjoy, and would spend much of the day feeling bored and frustrated, but with no motivation to do anything else. Sometimes he would still be in his pyjamas when his wife got home from work. This made him feel even worse about himself, triggering more negative thoughts and reinforcing his low mood.
>
> When Len started to focus on rebuilding structure into his days, he noticed very positive changes. He found that if he got up and had showered, shaved and dressed before breakfast (even if he didn't feel like it), then he was much more likely to pop out for a walk to the shops or around the park when he had finished his breakfast. As he did this he felt an improvement in his mood. He felt happier to stop and talk to neighbours when he saw them and gradually started to feel more motivated to build up his activity over the week.

Pleasure and achievement

There may be things that you are no longer able to do because of your health. We have met people who have had to give up certain interests and hobbies because of their condition and this can be extremely frustrating and upsetting. Part of adjusting to your condition is thinking creatively about how you can remain engaged in the things that interest you and are important to you, even if this is not in the same way as before.

When people feel down and their motivation is low, they tend gradually to stop doing things that would have previously given them pleasure or a sense of purpose and achievement. The less you do, the more time you have to sit and ruminate and get caught up in negative thinking, and the worse you will feel. Typically, if you are able to spend time doing things that give you *pleasure* and a sense of *achievement*, then it is likely that your day will feel more fulfilling. If you keep this up, it can lead to an improvement in how you feel. The following technique will help guide you in how to increase your activity levels in a helpful way.

1 First of all, measure your levels of activity in a week using an activity schedule (see Len's example in Table 6.1, overleaf). Fill in what you are doing at various points in your day. Once you have filled in the activity, rate it on a scale of 0 to 5 according to how pleasurable it is (P) and how much of a sense of achievement it gives you (A). For example, if you went to meet a friend for a cup of coffee, it might have been very pleasurable (4 out of 5) but did not make you feel you had achieved much (2 out of 5). Alternatively, if you did a spring clean of the kitchen, it might not have been enjoyable at all (0 out of 5) but you might have felt a strong sense of achievement afterwards (5 out of 5).

When Len completed an activity schedule he was shocked at how little he was doing and could see that the way he was spending his time gave him virtually no sense of pleasure or achievement. He could see that on his days at home on his own he would spend time ruminating on negative thoughts in front of the TV, and this was making his mood lower. Len also reflected on the impact of his inactivity on his negative thinking about himself (e.g. 'I am worthless', 'I have no purpose'), which made him feel even worse. He also noticed that on the days that his wife was at home and encouraged him to get up, shower and go out and see people – even though he never wanted to do this – it was better for him than doing nothing.

Table 6.1 Len's activity schedule

	Monday	Tuesday	Wednesday	Thursday	Friday	Saturday	Sunday
Morning	Breakfast Watch TV A 1/5, P 2/5	Breakfast Watch TV A 1/5, P 2/5	Breakfast Watch TV A 1/5, P 1/5	Breakfast Read newspaper A 3/5, P 2/5	Breakfast Watch TV A 1/5, P 1/5	Shower and shave Breakfast A 4/5, P 4/5	Shower and shave Breakfast A 3/5, P 3/5
Afternoon	Watch TV Unload dishwasher A 3/5, P 1/5	Watch TV A 1/5, P 2/5	Watch TV A 1/5, P 1/5	Watch film A 1/5, P 3/5	Watch TV A 1/5, P 1/5	Son and grandchildren visit A 2/5, P 4/5	Shopping with wife A 4/5, P 3/5
Evening	Watch TV Cook dinner A 3/5, P 2/5	Watch TV Take-away dinner A 1/5, P 2/5	Daughter visits for dinner A 2/5, P 3/5	Watch TV Take-away dinner A 1/5, P 2/5	To pub for drink with wife A 2/5, P 3/5	Dinner Read book A 2/5, P 3/5	Cook dinner Watch TV A 3/5, P 2/5

2 Next, write a list of everything that currently gives you a sense of pleasure or has done in the past – and a sense of achievement. For example, you may not have swum for years but you may remember that you used to really enjoy swimming and found it very relaxing. If you get stuck here, it can be helpful to ask people close to you to help you.

3 Select some of these activities and start to plan them into your week. You can use the same timetable as in Table 6.1 and write in some of these activities ahead of time. Sometimes you will need to make adjustments to the things that you previously enjoyed so that they work for you now.

As you can see from his activity schedule four weeks later (Table 6.2, overleaf), Len gradually planned his week so that he had a good mix of these activities each day. He also found that even activities he thought he would have to abandon could still be enjoyed with some adaptation. For example, he had always loved sailing on the local lake but had been told by his doctor that he needed to wait several months for his chest to heal before doing this again. Len realized that he missed not just the sailing but also being outdoors and seeing his friends. He went to visit the lake and to meet his friends and watch the sailing twice a week. He also helped out where he could. While he did feel frustrated that he was not out sailing, he recognized that being at the lake felt much better than being at home doing nothing. He also increased his physical exercise, going for regular walks and swimming, which he said was making him feel better both physically and emotionally. He also ensured that he saw more of his friends and family, which helped him to shift his focus more on to others and away from himself and his problems.

Physical exercise

Plenty of evidence shows that increasing your levels of physical activity can significantly improve your mood. Your ability to undertake such activity will depend on your physical condition, although doctors recommend at least some physical activity for most conditions. Physical activity improves energy levels, which in turn improves motivation and mood. Speak to your doctor about which activity is safe for you personally, and at what intensity. Once you have established this, we would strongly recommend building up your activity levels slowly and safely.

Table 6.2 Len's activity schedule four weeks later

	Monday	Tuesday	Wednesday	Thursday	Friday	Saturday	Sunday
Morning	Shower and shave Breakfast Walk in park A 3/5, P 2/5	Shower and shave Breakfast Walk in park A 3/5, P 2/5	Shower and shave Breakfast Walk in park A 3/5, P 2/5	Breakfast Read newspaper Tidy kitchen A 3/5, P 2/5	Shower and shave Breakfast Read newspaper Do washing A 3/5, P 2/5	Shower and shave Breakfast at cafe Walk with wife A 3/5, P 4/5	Shower and shave Breakfast Walk with wife A 3/5, P 4/5
Afternoon	Go swimming A 4/5, P 3/5	Sailing club A 3/5, P 4/5	Watch TV A 1/5, P 2/5	Sailing club A 4/5, P 4/5	Collect grandchildren from school A 4/5, P 4/5	Watch football match on TV A 1/5, P 3/5	Son and grandchildren visit A 2/5, P 4/5
Evening	Watch TV Cook dinner A 3/5, P 2/5	To pub for drink with wife A 2/5, P 3/5	Daughter visits for dinner A 2/5, P 3/5	Watch TV Cook dinner A 3/5, P 2/5	To pub for drink with wife A 2/5, P 3/5	Dinner Read book A 2/5, P 3/5	Cook dinner Watch TV A 3/5, P 2/5

Contact with others

When you feel low in mood, it is common to want to withdraw from others. However, this is very unhelpful. We are social beings and do not tend to do well in isolation, even if withdrawing is what we feel tempted to do. Planning regular contact with people in your week is very important, particularly if you live alone.

2 Challenging negative thinking

It is very natural to experience negative thoughts if you are diagnosed with a medical problem. Some of the thoughts might be accurate and appropriate. When we feel low in mood, though, we are likely to think much more negatively. As mentioned earlier, it is as if we have lenses that mean that all we can see are the bad and negative, and we can miss the positive and good going on around us. For this reason, if you take all your thoughts at face value and get caught up in them, then you will feel really terrible. In addition, unhelpful patterns of rumination can eat up a great deal of time and can lead to feeling very low indeed.

Because we know that much negative thinking is biased thinking and can be unrealistic, one approach to negative thoughts is to challenge them.

> Marian, 35, was diagnosed with breast cancer. She had surgery to remove one of her breasts and believed that her partner would henceforth no longer be attracted to her. She felt very low in mood and started to withdraw from her partner, spending less time with him in the house and avoiding any physical intimacy with him. Marian had patterns of rumination in which she would catastrophize (think about all the worst possible outcomes). Her thoughts tended to follow this pattern: 'My partner will not find me attractive any more and will probably leave me', 'No one will ever find me attractive again', 'I will be single for the rest of my life', 'I won't ever have children and this will make me extremely unhappy', 'I will be alone and miserable for ever'.

Here you can see that the longer Marian followed her train of thought, the more desperate her thoughts got and the worse she felt. She was advised to challenge her initial thought that 'my partner will no longer be attracted to me and will leave me'.

Techniques for challenging negative thoughts

First, identify some of the negative thoughts that tend to go round and round your head. When you have written them down, go through them one by one. For each thought, ask yourself the questions outlined in Chapter 3 (page 26) when we encouraged you to challenge your unhelpful health beliefs. You can also try to develop more helpful alternative thoughts using the process outlined in Chapter 5 (page 46) when challenging your anxious thoughts.

> Marian was very interested to see that she did not believe her original thoughts as deeply after she had done this exercise. She recognized that she did not have any evidence to suggest that her partner would leave her, and indeed that there was quite a bit of evidence to suggest that he was still committed to her. This didn't mean that she didn't have the thoughts again, but she did not tend to get stuck in such unhelpful patterns of catastrophizing.

When you have identified some alternative thoughts, try to put this new way of thinking into practice. You may notice that your negative thoughts are still triggered, but the more you step back and notice when they are there, the easier it will become to replace those negative thoughts with your more balanced alternative thoughts. Sometimes it is helpful to have a list of common negative thoughts and helpful alternatives to refer back to if you notice you are getting stuck in your negative patterns of thinking again.

What if the negative thoughts are true?

Of course, in some instances you will have negative and upsetting thoughts that are not biased and are potentially absolutely true and realistic. In the context of physical illness this can happen because there is often real and bad news to adjust to. In these instances, challenging them would not be helpful.

> Jennifer was diagnosed with heart failure when she was 40 years old. She was told by her doctors that while they could manage her condition and symptoms well, they could not reverse the condition and it was likely significantly to shorten her life span. Jennifer felt extremely depressed. She thought deeply about what she would miss out on if she died younger than she had anticipated. She wondered if she might miss her children growing up, or if she might miss having grandchildren. This inevitably led to withdrawal and rumination.

For Jennifer, sadly, such thoughts were not unrealistic. Indeed, her fears of missing people and events that were important to her were justified. However, this did not mean that she could not improve how she felt. While Jennifer did not challenge the *truth* of her thoughts, she still recognized that sitting in her room and focusing on these thoughts for hours at a time was not helping her at all. Jennifer realized that getting caught in patterns of rumination was not only making her very upset, but was also making her miss out on the time that she *did* have with her family. She therefore developed mindfulness skills to help reduce the impact of these thoughts on her. The same strategies are helpful, whether for letting go of worry or dealing with unhelpful negative thoughts, and we encourage you to revisit the techniques outlined in Chapter 5 (pages 46–7) and let go of your unhelpful negative thoughts.

3 Problem-solving

When we feel depressed, our motivation to address and face issues can be considerably reduced. It is common to feel hopeless and helpless about your ability to solve a problem such as financial issues. Sometimes people take an avoidant approach and try to pretend something isn't happening. Other people worry and worry about what might go wrong but do not do anything about it. Both of these strategies tend to lead to the actual 'problem' getting worse and the individual feeling worse as a result.

Try the following steps towards active problem-solving:

1 Identify the problem you want to work on.
2 Think of as many ways to solve the problem as you can.
3 Work out what solutions on your list seem to be the best. You can consider the pros and cons of different possible solutions and use this to rank the solutions in order of preference.
4 Pick the solution that you think has the best balance.
5 Work out all the small steps that are required to achieve this solution.
6 Put the first small step into action and review how it goes.
7 Continue this process until the problem is solved or helped, or until it is clear that there are no more possible solutions.

Holding on to hope

It is helpful to remember that human beings have a remarkable threshold to withstand suffering and that even in the hardest of situations we do still have some choices available to us. Over history, accounts from people in the most horrendous of circumstances have shown us that we can still feel connected to others and take pleasure in small things in our lives.

Trevor is 60 years old and has advanced pancreatic cancer. He is in pain and it is difficult for him to move around. He has been told that he will probably not live longer than three months. Of course, Trevor and his family are devastated by this news. Trevor does not want to die and finds it unspeakably upsetting to think of leaving his wife, children and grandchildren behind. He feels very sad and very angry at times and gets very frustrated by how little he can do for himself. His natural reaction was to brood over how unfair it was and to dwell on several very understandable negative thoughts. One day, following a conversation with one of his oldest friends, Trevor realized that he did have a choice about how he approached these coming months. He could either spend them dwelling on negative thoughts, shutting other people out and feeling depressed, or he could try to make the most of the time he had. Trevor started to notice and treasure small pleasures, and his family worked hard to identify meaningful events that he could experience, despite his pain and incapacitation:

• Trevor's grandchildren came to visit twice a week and he would read to them.
• His family brought old photos down from the attic and Trevor would help his wife sort through these for an hour a day.
• Trevor's son made him a playlist of all his favourite music from the 1960s to listen to.
• They would leave his bedroom window open. Even when it was quite cold Trevor enjoyed the feeling of fresh air on his face.
• His family arranged for him to meet their local vicar twice a week. He found these conversations helpful as he felt he could talk about death and dying and his beliefs about what would happen to him after death.
• Trevor and his family had open, honest conversations with his healthcare team in which he was able to talk about his fears concerning his final days and what they could put in place for this time. While these were very upsetting and difficult conversations, Trevor found having a plan reassuring.

Trevor found the last few months of his life more peaceful and more enjoyable than he ever expected. This does not mean that he did not feel frightened, angry, in pain and extremely upset, but he also felt loved, he felt connected to those around him, he felt useful and he felt grateful for everyone's kindness.

When you are trying to hold on to hope, what you personally find helpful will be very individual to you. So you need to find sources of strength that fit with you and your life and beliefs and interests. Here are some general ideas that can help maintain a sense of hope:

- focusing on what you can enjoy in your life as it is now;
- focusing on what you are able to do;
- making an effort to see people you have not seen for a while;
- keeping an open dialogue with your healthcare team;
- going to your place of worship;
- praying;
- meditating.

Severe depression and suicidal thoughts

Some people experience very entrenched and powerful experiences of depression, which can escalate into thoughts about not wanting to live any more and even overt thoughts of suicide. If this is you, we recommend that you speak with your GP or someone in your specialist care team as soon as possible. Don't be put off by fearing that it's too difficult a topic, or that no one can help. On the contrary, your healthcare team will most certainly have spoken to people who have felt a similar way and will be able to advise you. Please also see the final chapter in this book for 'when this book is not enough'.

7

Managing self-esteem
in the context of illness

Many people struggle with shifts in their self-esteem in the context of changes that occur with the onset of illness. This can include changing roles, changes in your ability and appearance, and the impact of your condition on work and your social life. Lowered self-esteem can further exacerbate experiences of low mood and anxiety. This chapter aims to normalize these difficulties and provide cognitive behavioural strategies to help protect your self-esteem in the face of these challenges.

Most people experience self-doubt at some point in their lives, whether through entrenched low self-esteem or other factors. Some people, for example, have a specific aspect of themselves that they dislike, such as their appearance, manners, attitude, social status or ability to carry out certain tasks or master specific activities. Other people may dislike themselves in a general way and therefore lack confidence in many situations. Low self-esteem can affect people's thoughts, feelings, behaviours and relationships.

Common symptoms of low self-esteem
Cognitive/thinking symptoms
- *Self-criticism* This may include thoughts of not coping with your illness or thinking that you have burdened your family or friends.
- *Self-doubt* You may doubt or question whether you can cope with your condition or if you ever will be able to function normally again. Some people may also question their physical appearance, work identity or relationships.
- *Discounting the positive* Low self-esteem often leads people to discount or ignore their strengths and positive attributes. You may find that you focus on what you perceive as your weakness instead, for example, of allowing yourself to recognize the bravery you show when trying to manage your health problems.

- *Self-consciousness* A sense of being over-aware of oneself during social encounters is often due to a fear of being negatively evaluated by other people. You may, for example, worry more about your appearance, saying the wrong thing, talking too much about your health or burdening other people with your problems. You may also be self-conscious about other people treating you differently because of your condition.
- *Self-blame* Low self-esteem can cause you to blame yourself, even if an event is not directly associated with you. For example, you may blame yourself for having developed the condition in the first place: 'If I had looked after my health better, I might not have developed my illness.' You may also blame yourself for not having visited your doctor sooner or think that you should have been more vigilant towards symptoms of ill health.

Feelings

These feelings are indicators of low self-esteem:

- guilt
- shame
- frustration
- anger (often directed towards oneself)
- worthlessness
- sadness
- anxiety.

Behaviours

- *Pleasing behaviours* People with low self-confidence may try to please other people, sometimes at the expense of their own needs. You may find that you are giving in to your children's demands more often after becoming unwell, or you may feel less inclined to let other people know if they have upset you or are placing unreasonable demands on you.
- *Working too hard* We are all guilty of taking on too much work or responsibility at some point in our lives. People with low self-esteem may fall into this trap by frequently agreeing or volunteering to take on extra work or responsibilities, both at work and in their personal lives. You may, for example, find that you are trying to do too much during the day, leaving you feeling very tired. This may be because you are struggling to adapt to the limitations of your

condition, or because you are trying to reassure other people close to you that you can cope.

- *Avoidance* Some people with low self-esteem may also avoid taking on new challenges or seeking opportunities at work or at home through a fear of failing or of not being good enough to complete the task in hand. You may, for example, find that you stop volunteering to help out at your children's local school or you decline a promotion at work because you fear it may jeopardize your health.
- *Withdrawal from other people* Low self-esteem can sometimes lead people to withdraw from friends, colleagues or family members. You may feel that you are burdening others or that they feel sorry for you because of your illness. Withdrawing from other people can perpetuate feelings of isolation, loneliness and low self-worth. Becoming isolated can lead to further issues such as anxiety and low mood.

Lisa was frequently asked by colleagues to take on additional tasks at work, despite being incredibly busy with balancing her own workload with chronic migraines. She did not want colleagues to think of her as 'lazy' or 'unhelpful'. She stayed late in the office most days and would often bring work home. This had the effect of making her immediately feel less stressed about the prospect of being disliked by her colleagues, but the increased workload led to more migraines. She eventually became exhausted and had to take frequent time off work through being bedridden with severe migraine. The problem was that Lisa never dared to say 'no' to her colleagues. She therefore did not get the chance to discover that most people would approve of her regardless of whether she refused to help out with their work. In the end her migraines worsened and she had to take time off work, which obviously impacted negatively on her colleagues, anyway.

Other common behaviours of this type include suppressing your own needs to please others, over-thinking social situations and 'going overboard' to accommodate other people.

Being unwell can cause changes, some transient and others more long lasting. Sometimes people may be required to renegotiate their occupation, social network or the particular role they play within the family, with partners or friends or at work.

Many of us measure our worth and the worth of others by achievements. Successes in particular aspects of our lives, such as parenting, in our relationships or in our careers, may reflect what we consider to be important achievements. When illness forces changes in these or other areas that define us, we may begin to feel worthless. Parents may find that having to adapt or withdraw from their supportive and protective role in a family is a particularly heavy burden and one that challenges their sense of 'worth'. Associated with this may be feelings of guilt for exposing our children to difficulties. Being unwell can have an impact on capability, which in turn affects our identity and self-esteem.

> Karen was in her early 30s when she had a stroke that left her paralysed on the left side of her face. This made a visual change to her facial features, which Karen found difficult to accept. She tried a number of medical and plastic surgeries to help lift the left side of her mouth and eye but she did not feel confident about the way she looked. She would often wear big sunglasses in an attempt to cover her face and she also tended to hide her mouth behind her hand when speaking to other people. She felt ashamed, unattractive and different. Karen gradually became increasingly insecure and felt self-conscious even in the presence of her partner. About two years after the stroke, Karen and her husband had twins. Becoming a parent made Karen start to appreciate the many positive qualities she possessed as a strong-willed mother and wife who had overcome an acute health problem.

Karen learned to be confident by reminding herself that she was much more than her facial visible difference. Most of us have something about ourselves we wish we could change (appearance, age, nationality or personality, for example), whether this is visible or hidden. The arrival of the twins allowed Karen to focus on a different aspect of herself where she could build confidence by caring for her children.

> Jax, a 27-year-old musician, suffered from erectile dysfunction. This had been a problem since he had a car accident when he was 14. He had not been able to have sexual intercourse until he sought medical treatment at age 26. Up until then Jax had felt so embarrassed about his problem that he avoided dating girls. He would often question himself, 'Am I not man enough to have sex?', 'What is wrong with me?' and 'I must be weird since I am not capable of doing what my friends are doing.' It took Jax a long time to be able to be intimate with his girlfriend following medical treatment. When he did, Jax discovered to his surprise that he was able to let go of the shame and self-consciousness he had felt for so long. He did not mind having to take the medication prior to having sexual intercourse. Instead, there was a sense of relief and joy over the ability to be able to experiment sexually with his girlfriend.

Years of shame and anxiety about having erectile dysfunction had prevented Jax from seeking medical help. Having been with his girlfriend for over two years, Jax realized that she was attracted as much to his personality as to his sexual characteristics. With his girlfriend's support, Jax was able to confront his problem by seeking medical help and started to build his self-esteem. This allowed him to focus on things that he could do and to enjoy them. He was able to demonstrate confidence in living with and managing his condition.

Building self-esteem using cognitive behavioural therapy (CBT)

Any condition, whether non-life-threatening or terminal, can affect our beliefs about the world, ourselves and the people around us. We may begin to question beliefs that we thought were fundamental to our identity, and to re-evaluate the basic ideas we have about living and indeed about who we are as individuals. Some people look for spiritual help in their search for understanding and meaning. Some may find solace in learning about approaches that they might not have once considered to be options for themselves. Others may question or even renounce their religion in the face of their own health problems or of problems experienced by someone close to them.

The impact on beliefs can also be subtle. An ill parent, for example, may feel his confidence and certainty about his role as a parent is disrupted by the changes he is going through. A dedicated career person who has worked hard all her life to be successful and wealthy may question the point of these achievements in the face of a medical issue. In the most direct way, health problems can change what we believe in and what we believe about ourselves. The independent, brave, stalwart character you thought you would always be may be elusive when you are unwell, or may come and go alongside the changes in your symptoms.

As introduced in Chapter 1, CBT helps people to identify the unhelpful patterns of thinking and behaving that we get caught in and outlines strategies to break these unhelpful cycles and develop new and more helpful ones. As has been described above, when people have low self-esteem, there are particular patterns of thinking and behaving that contribute to, maintain and exacerbate feeling negative about themselves.

Leila dedicated most of her time to researching diets and medical treatments to improve her health. She would spend hours on the internet every evening, despite being reassured by her doctor that her health was improving. Leila had a history of low self-esteem, having been bullied in high school for several years. For six months she saw a psychologist who helped her recognize how the over-focus on other people, her work or her boyfriend might be an attempt to give her a legitimate excuse not to attend to her own needs. Her low self-worth would sometimes cause her to think, 'I am not worth it', 'Why bother about myself?' This unfortunately made Leila more prone to focusing on external issues, as they distracted her from having to consider her own needs. Leila was eventually able to recognize how the focus, time and effort dedicated to researching her health perpetuated her low self-worth because it reduced her capacity to attend to her own needs.

Ed, on the other hand, avoided seeing people, including friends and family. He often cancelled or refused to commit to social activities. Having developed insulin-dependent diabetes, Ed felt that his social life would never be the same. His diet and alcohol consumption had been seriously restricted by his condition and Ed therefore thought that his friends would perceive him as 'boring' and 'weak'. He became increasingly isolated, lonely and sad.

The life-balance diary

Keeping a life-balance diary could help you to improve your self-esteem by planning more satisfying activities; Ed found that it helped him to recognize how withdrawal from his friends and family had affected his mood and self-esteem. A life-balance diary is simply a way of planning your life so that you dedicate necessary time to caring for yourself while juggling daily demands from others. It is important that you fill the diary with activities that you enjoy and that are important to you, and for this reason we cannot be prescriptive about what to do. How much to include also depends on you: you may find that your activity level tends to drop during periods of poor health and increase when you feel better.

When starting the life-balance diary you may just wish to monitor your activities for the first week. This will allow you to reflect on how you spend your time and to consider what you would like to change. The following questions may help:

- Am I striking a balance between spending time on others, on daily activities and on myself?
- Are there any activities that I enjoy more than others? What area do I naturally spend most of my time on?

- Am I withdrawing from others? If so, why? Who do I feel more comfortable seeing (specific friend, family member, etc.)?
- How much time am I spending on daily activities? Do I feel bad about other people supporting me? Is there a part of me that is trying to do too much? If so, why?
- Am I trying too hard to be independent because I feel so dependent on other people for my health or want to prove that I can cope?
- Can I outsource more of the daily tasks to release more time dedicated to my family or myself?
- Am I doing too much for other people?

The second step is to start planning ahead, using the questions above to help you identify suitable activities. You could plan up to three days in advance so that you already have a structure when you wake up. This may reduce the risk that indecisiveness or low mood in the morning prevents you from being active during the day. You can use the activity planning schedule outlined and discussed in Chapter 6 as a basis for a life-balance diary (see Tables 6.1 and 6.2, pages 58 and 60).

Identifying personal qualities

People with low self-esteem may find it difficult to identify their positive qualities, or they may quickly discount their positive attributes and focus more on what they perceive to be their negative qualities.

> Joanna was concerned that she was unable to take her kids to school because her medication prevented her from driving. She ignored the fact that she would always get up in the morning to ensure the children had breakfast and were washed and dressed. Joanna paid too much attention to what she could not do and therefore failed to note the many things she was still able to do for her family.

Take care not to fall into the trap of constantly criticizing and questioning yourself. You may well have thoughts such as 'Other people do a much better job than me', 'I am not completely satisfied with my performance' and 'I must try harder.' These statements may lead you to ignore or discount your positive qualities, so that you waste your energy on tasks you can't do or end up feeling inferior to others. The following questions may be able to help you become more aware of positive qualities:

- What are the qualities I like about myself?
- What have I achieved that I am proud of? (You may wish to start

by thinking back to your adolescent years and then working through to the present. Examples of positive achievements could include passing exams at school, getting a job, going to university, doing charity work, caring for a friend or family member, helping someone else out when they needed it, holding down a job, working out on a regular basis, balancing work and your health, being in a relationship, having children and so on.)

- Is there anything that I have done earlier this week or today that was positive? (This could include letting someone pass in front of you while queuing to pay for groceries, talking to and sharing your experiences with a fellow patient in the hospital, making your partner a nice meal, saying good morning to the neighbour, giving up your seat to a pregnant lady on the bus, and so on.)
- Did I offer any nice comments or feedback to people around me?
- Did I ensure that I got enough rest today so that I had more energy when I spent time with my friend?
- Is there anything else I can think of that I do which is positive? (This includes writing emails to friends, thinking positive thoughts about others and yourself, letting go of worries and focusing on one day at a time.)
- If I asked a friend to comment on my positive qualities, what would he or she say?
- What negative qualities do I *not* have? (For example, are you the kind of person who is deliberately mean to other people? Do you enjoy putting other people down?)
- What type of positive qualities do I admire in other people? (It may be helpful to make a list of these. When you have done so, try to think about whether you possess any of these qualities yourself. If not, think about how you can develop these.)

Keeping a diary of your positive qualities like the one in Table 7.1 (overleaf) may help you to be more aware of them.

Try to document as many situations as you can on a daily basis. It is absolutely fine to miss a couple of days if you feel unwell or are too busy to make entries in the diary. The best thing to do is to follow your own pace and do as much as you can when you feel like it. It would be beneficial to keep the diary going over a period of perhaps six months or more so that you can train yourself to become better at spotting positive qualities.

Table 7.1 Positive qualities diary

Situation	My positive quality	Evidence to support the positive quality
A man asking for directions to a particular department in the hospital	Helpful Caring	I directed him to the information desk
Returned to work	Likeable Valuable member of the team	Colleagues had bought me gifts and seemed genuinely happy that I am back
Finding a costume for my child's school play	Good mum	My son was pleased with his costume He looked very confident during the school play

Identifying and challenging negative thoughts about yourself

As we have already mentioned earlier in this chapter, people with low self-esteem may have critical and negative thoughts about themselves that can maintain low self-esteem. A good way of picking up on such unhelpful thoughts is to keep a journal of critical thoughts and think about how to replace these with a kinder, less critical way of evaluating yourself.

> Ben's wife pointed out that she thought he should contribute more around the house now that his health was on the mend. This immediately made Ben think that his wife saw him as useless and lazy. An alternative explanation to the wife's comment may be that she wanted to help and thought that it was important for Ben to engage with daily household chores to regain a sense of normality and structure.

Keeping a written record of self-critical or anxiety-provoking thoughts can be an effective way of making you more aware of negative thinking patterns that stop you from feeling better about yourself. In order to challenge your negative thoughts about yourself, we encourage you to revisit the exercises in Chapter 3 for challenging unhelpful health beliefs (page 26).

Although this chapter has focused on helping you build your self-esteem, it is important to emphasize that very few people are ever 100 per cent satisfied with themselves. As humans we have many qualities, some of which we like and some of which we do not like. This is completely normal and part of the unique composition of personal qualities that makes us into who we are as individuals. The key is to learn to accept who you are, the things you can and can't do. None of us is perfect no matter how much we may strive to change ourselves, and it is therefore important to work with what you have got rather than to focus too much on what you perceive to be your flaws.

8

Talking to friends and family

It is well established that perceived social support has a major influence on reducing anxiety, depression and stress. We know that this is also true in the context of impaired health. Telling others in the family about your physical condition is usually a big challenge for several reasons. It signals the potential for changes in the family's structure, roles and relationships, patterns of care and support, and the possibility (and sometimes too the inevitability) of actual loss, as well as indirect changes in other family members. There is also the possibility of having to cancel or postpone one's own plans and future aspirations. An example is a son who is giving up his football practice to take his mother to dialysis. Or maybe a husband is giving up his study at home for his wife, who is being treated for emphysema and needs more space for the medical equipment she needs to manage her breathing difficulties.

Disclosure

Disclosure of illness – the act of telling others the nature of the medical problem and what it means – is not always a carefully planned event. Sometimes it comes to light because a child has seen a letter from the clinic or a partner overhears a telephone discussion with a doctor. At these times, you may be confronted with questions which need to be answered either in a completely honest way or with the minimum of information in order to begin to build up knowledge and understanding over time. Disclosure is usually *selective*. This means that we do not normally tell everyone everything at once. Most people tell only selected family and friends at first and may only give limited information at this time. This may be because there is only limited information about the condition that is available at the time. It may also be because you are 'testing' others to see how they react and cope with some understanding before telling them more, or before sharing with them more difficult and possibly more emotionally painful aspects of what lies ahead. Disclosure is therefore also *incremental*.

Felicity had been trying to conceive for over two years when she and her husband went to see a specialist. During one of her examinations, the doctor told Felicity that she had primary ovarian insufficiency (POI) and was therefore unable to conceive. He suggested that they could try IVF. Felicity initially felt ashamed, thinking that she should be able to conceive naturally. She ignored messages from close friends and family asking her how she and her husband were doing. Felicity could not bear telling them her news and she therefore decided to gradually open up to close friends and family. She started by telling her mum, who was supportive and empathetic. The positive and encouraging reaction from her mother helped Felicity feel more at ease when telling the rest of her family.

Felicity felt apprehensive about telling her friends and family about her condition and especially its impact on the couple's ability to conceive. How a person chooses to disclose medical issues to family and friends is essentially a personal matter. Here are some loose guidelines on things you may want to consider:

- Consider how people will react and understand that this will depend on what and how you tell them.
- Choose whom you want, or need, to tell.
- Plan when and where you will tell people (avoid noisy public places and times when there are children around or there is little time for further discussion).
- Think whether there is anything you want from the person: if so, ask directly.
- Emotional expression is normal. People should expect you to be 'real' and display normal emotions and feelings. Encourage these in other people.
- When disclosing, first tell the facts and what you know. Then tell what is still being investigated and what is unknown, and then tell the person how you feel.
- Consider disclosure as part of a longer-term process: you don't have to say everything at once. You may need to tell more at another time.

The way people break the news will also vary. Some people prefer to tell others face to face, whereas others prefer to speak on the phone. Some may wish to inform friends and family via text message or email, while others just prefer to let other people tell friends and family about their problems. There is no right or wrong way of disclosing your health condition. What works for one individual and his or her family may not work for another. The best advice is to do what seems and feels right for you at the time.

> Raymond chose to disclose his diagnosis of cancer via a text message to his close friends. This was after he had broken the news in person to his family.
>
> Raymond's wife was eight months pregnant when he was diagnosed with terminal brain cancer. This was their first child. His main concern was to secure the future of their daughter and his wife. Raymond found it difficult to tell his friends about his situation. After he had discussed it with his wife, they both decided that Raymond should send a text message to his friends:
>
> > There is no easy way to tell you our sad news. I have terminal brain cancer. They don't know how long I have left but the doctors estimate anything between one and five years. I am OK. My main concern is to secure the future of my wife and our little girl. I know they will be fine with your help. I will be in touch soon.

Managing other people's reactions

People around you will react differently to your news. Even close friends may find it hard to know what to say to you. They may avoid seeing you or speaking about your health, a reaction that can be very upsetting. The majority of your friends and colleagues are likely to be well-meaning, but not all will fully understand what you are experiencing unless they themselves have been unwell.

> Valerie, a 30-year-old architect, was diagnosed with chronic fatigue. Her family and friends were all very supportive when she first told them the news. Work was also understanding and allowed her to reduce her working hours for two months, as requested by her doctor. Valerie continued to come down with various cold and flu-like illnesses over the next six months. She was constantly tired and spent a great deal of time in bed, resting or sleeping. This led her to take time off work and she also had to cancel most of her social engagements. As the time elapsed, some of the people around her became less patient and more frustrated with her condition. Valerie eventually saw a counsellor who helped her understand why some family members and friends found it difficult to accept her condition. She came to understand that the condition itself,

chronic fatigue, may be a complex one that is not so easy for other people to understand, especially as there are no visual indications of physical illness.

Your family and loved ones may be in emotional turmoil too, bewildered and anxious as they try to adjust to your illness. It is important to remember that some people will not know what to say or do. They may be afraid, embarrassed or confused. Some may rally and be supportive; others may mean well but upset you with their suggestions and ideas of what you should do; yet others may simply disappear, finding it all too much to bear emotionally, and so withdrawing to protect themselves from loss. If they don't literally stop visiting, they may minimize the gravity of your condition or refuse to acknowledge the seriousness of your challenges. Sadly, the effect can be a negative one, leaving you feeling rejected and isolated.

Some people are changeable. You may find that a family member is initially supportive but gradually finds it more difficult to deal with your condition as time elapses. Conversely, friends may initially withdraw because they struggle to cope, only to come back when they are ready to deal with the situation.

It may make sense to differentiate between the family impact of a short or acute health problem and the impact of a lifelong chronic condition, as these tend to lead to different emotional reactions. Acute illness may in the short term lead to very intense expressed emotions. A good example is when a wife discovers that her husband has had a heart attack, or when a brother finds out that his sister has had an accident and is in intensive care. A lifelong chronic condition, on the other hand, may lead to curtailing life's ambitions and bring irritability and resentment. This was the case with Valerie, who suffered from chronic fatigue. This distinction may also be important when attempting to understand the impact these emotional reactions may have on the person concerned.

Valerie, for example, felt that her family and friends were initially supportive but as time elapsed they became less patient. This may have made her feel upset, frustrated or even guilty. Likewise, the wife whose husband had a heart attack may initially experience intense feelings of fear, shock and disbelief, which may lead the husband to worry about her and blame himself for causing her so much pain.

Relationships with loved ones may need to adapt; roles within the family often shift. Depending on your diagnosis and treatment regime, you may need to come to terms with stopping work for a period or changing some other aspects of your lifestyle. For some, where a medical problem is terminal and nature is taking its course, these limitations and changes may be considerable and permanent. Some people find that if the health condition or its treatment affects their body and the way they feel about themselves, it can have an effect on their intimate relationships. We explore this further in our chapter on self-esteem issues (see Chapter 7).

Remember that just as you hold health beliefs (discussed in Chapter 3) based on your experiences and your family stories, so will those around you. The health beliefs that your family and friends hold are likely to affect how they respond to your health condition.

The following questions may help you to explore the beliefs that may guide you concerning your family's way of dealing with the news of your illness.

- What views do your family hold about modern medicine in general? Perhaps you come from a family who worry about getting sick and visit the doctor often just to make sure they are in good health. On the other hand, your family may hold the view that you should just dust yourself off and get on with it; they may be less inclined to seek medical help, even if symptoms are worrying. What are your views?
- Is there a conflict between your views and those of family members?
- Do members of your family or people you are close to have particular views or attitudes towards you and your condition?
- Do they express these attitudes towards you and your health condition? They might suggest, either explicitly or by their actions, that 'it's your own fault' or that 'you should have listened to me'. Their reactions, such as withdrawal from you, being judgemental or being afraid to be around you, may reflect some of the deeper feelings and fears that they have.

These questions may not be easy or straightforward to answer. As we discussed in the section on health beliefs, these may have an effect on how you and your family initially understand your condition, what you think your treatment can do for you, the strength of your relationships with loved ones, as well as with doctors, and your approaches to self-care. Thinking about what your family and friends believe about being unwell may help you to understand better their behaviour and reactions to your condition.

Organizing continuing support

A final point to consider is how you can organize family support. These are guidelines only, as the way that works for you is essentially unique, depending on the nature of your condition, your social network, your circumstances and your personal characteristics.

- Think of what you need and want from people. Draw up a list and think in terms of healthcare issues, practical support, financial concerns, emotional issues and, if relevant, support for children.
- Ask people directly! Waiting for them to offer could prove frustrating and disappointing. Sometimes people are concerned that they will upset you further by offering to help. It may therefore be preferable and more rewarding to request help directly.
- Try to spread the demands around to different family members so as not to overburden any one person. If necessary, draw up a rota.
- Discuss your concerns with those whose help, though offered, doesn't seem to materialize. Don't let your disappointments fester.
- Try to remember to show your appreciation. This reinforces people's helping behaviour.

We recognize that for some people it is very difficult to ask for help. We all hold our own ideas and attitudes towards asking for and receiving support. If you find this particularly difficult it may help to imagine that you are in the position of your loved ones. If you thought that a friend or family member was struggling with coping with being unwell and needed more support, would you want her to suffer in silence or would you rather she asked you for help?

There is not a right or wrong way of telling other people about your health problems or organizing their support. Some people prefer to wait a while before feeling able to share their news, whereas others may want to talk about it the very same day. The way you choose to communicate your health condition to others is essentially an individual decision and will depend upon the preference, needs and wants you and your family or friends have.

The next chapter will look at how to make the most out of the support available from your medical team.

9

Making the most of support from your medical team

For most people, having a chronic or acute illness inevitably means developing a relationship with the healthcare system. For at least some of the time you will be a 'patient'.

Often a specific image will come to mind when you hear the term 'patient'. You may, as some people tell us, think that it makes you feel more dependent, disempowered, frail and separated from healthy, 'normal' people. 'Patient' seems to mean having different feelings from a healthy person.

Being designated a patient may change how you feel about yourself, and this in turn may affect how others see you. You may fear the term 'patient' as though in itself it is stigmatizing and debilitating. Even before you were diagnosed, you may have attended a hospital, perhaps on a one-off outpatient basis or to accompany someone to a clinical appointment, and will remember seeing rows of patients waiting for consultations. The experience of seeing people being processed and organized may have been unwelcome or even distasteful to you. Lengthy waits, uncomfortable seating, uncongenial surroundings, boredom, hunger and/or dehydration, fatigue, coupled with fear or anxiety, may well have left a negative impression.

In spite of all the advances in clinical medicine and healthcare which are so often in the news, being a patient in the twenty-first century still has its challenges and pressure points. Health settings now try to be more patient-centred and reflect the fact that treatment and care are more effective when patients are (or at least feel they are) partners in their own care. Medical school training these days teaches doctors to try to see the world through their patients' eyes and to empathize with what it is to be a patient. People are increasingly encouraged to be more involved in the way their health conditions are managed. They are supplied with information about their conditions, encouraged to join support groups, offered a choice of places where treatments are provided, and even invited to give feedback about their care.

Collaborative healthcare is increasingly common, both in GP practices and in specialist medical centres. Research demonstrates that where doctors and patients collaborate, quality of life improves, the number of clinic visits may be reduced, care costs can come down, and patients report improved satisfaction in their treatment and care, even if the outcome is not necessarily improved. This is a far cry from the older, more paternalistic, hierarchically arranged, doctor–patient relationship characterized by and satirized by Oscar Wilde in *The Importance of Being Earnest*:

ALGY	The doctors found out that Bunbury could not live, that is what I mean – so Bunbury died.
LADY BRACKNELL	He seems to have had great confidence in the opinion of his physicians.

'Doctor' comes from the Latin *docere* ('to instruct') and originally meant a teacher, by the Middle Ages coming to mean 'a learned person', while 'patient' derives from *patior* ('I suffer'). So the imbalance is there in the very terms 'doctor' and 'patient', and traditionally the expert, all-knowing doctor would have little time for dealing with the unique and specific concerns of a patient.

The internet provides a way for patients to become experts in their own conditions, and doctors now learn that treatment decisions should be made in a transparent way. Patients now, too, have access to their medical records, and some doctors copy correspondence to patients as a matter of course. These changes in the doctor–patient relationship and in patterns of communication between doctors and patients, as well as changes in the ambience of medical facilities, have altered what patients expect from consultations.

The other side to this is that there are now a number of important responsibilities that fall to us as patients. We are encouraged to be proactive and to understand our medical condition and the choices available to us. We need to navigate through the vast amount of health information now freely available to everyone. We must also try to look after our health and wellbeing, manage some of the physical and emotional impacts of our particular health condition and know how and whom to ask for help.

Finding and using information

Medical treatments advance rapidly in many areas and specialisms and new ones are being developed all the time. For example, we are learning more about the causes of cancer and what we can do to prevent it in the first place. Reports of ground-breaking discoveries, potential cures and new approaches to treatment – and even self-care – may raise hopes, but it is sometimes difficult to have a realistic sense of what they actually mean to you. Without some discussion with your doctor about your unique circumstances, it may be difficult to place this information in context and to think how best it applies to you. This, in turn affects how you are likely to feel about such information and advances.

When we are not well, information may take on additional importance. Our need to know what our own symptoms mean can make us vulnerable. While there is some truth to the old adage that 'knowledge is power', it has to be the *right* knowledge and it has to be used *appropriately*. If you are looking for information about your medical condition, here are some good places to start:

- *Your doctor* Consultations or appointments at the hospital or clinic provide an opportunity to ask questions and to clarify any issues you have about your condition. Clearly your starting point should be your GP, who will (depending on your condition) have referred you to a hospital specialist. These days all GPs have access to information about your condition, even if it is a rare one. They are unlikely – and do not need – to be experts in all aspects of the condition, but almost inevitably they will have come across it in the course of their training and experience and will certainly know where to access further information if needed. Your GP will be able to point you in the right direction, even if he or she is unable to address some of your questions.
- *Medical charities* Numerous medical charities in the UK provide specific information and support to people affected by a particular condition. Such organizations will have gathered and accrued vast amounts of information and experience in dealing with your condition. At the very least they will have written information, either in printed form or online, which will describe in layperson's terms the nature of your condition, possible treatments and what to expect. Hopefully there will also be some guidance on what you can do to cope better with your condition. Many such charities fund research into treatments and cures, and therefore it may be that members of the charity will be a good source of information about

what lies on the horizon as far as future treatments are concerned. They will also be able to direct you to specialist services and centres that deal with your specific medical condition.

- *Support organizations and groups* These provide a place to share experiences and learn new ways to cope with troubling feelings or symptoms. They also provide reassurance and enable you to improve your confidence in taking care of yourself. Many medical charities have local support groups across the country, so it may not be necessary to travel to large centres or key hospitals in order to access support. Some support may even be available in your own home, so it is important to ask if this will be possible for you.
- *The internet* An obvious source of information, this can be a gateway to support groups or forums and other resources specific to your health condition. You should of course be aware that the internet is a largely unregulated source of information, and you should also note that GPs and other health professionals will sometimes discourage you from searching out information about your condition in this way. In most instances this is not because they want to deter you from learning more in case this upsets you, but because the information may be unfiltered and therefore some advice, guidance or personal experiences may cause you needless harm and distress. It may be that the information reported applies to other groups of patients or some who have a different but related condition to your own.

Your healthcare experience

A range of professionals will be involved in your care. You may find it frustrating having to tell your story multiple times to different people, and it may be upsetting to realize that you are just one of several patients your medical professionals are seeing. At times you may feel let down; it is natural to expect healthcare providers to be omnipotent and to treat and cure us, to communicate well and clearly, to give sound guidance and to be empathetic and understanding at all times – but these professionals are only human and they are not going to be all these things all the time.

If you feel disappointment following a consultation, it is worth reflecting whether this might have been a one-off experience with a tired, stressed and overworked professional or whether it reflects a pattern in care. If the latter, it probably is time to find someone else to look after you.

As you build up a relationship with your healthcare team, you will learn the best way to communicate with each of them. Communication is a two-way process: a particular health professional will need to know what your symptoms are, how your medication is working and how you are coping. This person will need to examine you, observe you and at times obtain collateral or extended information about you from other sources, such as by seeking reports from another specialist or your GP. In the medical consultation, however, the information can only come from you. You, in turn, will rely on the medical professional's expertise to allay your fears, inform you of how your condition is affecting you now and is likely to affect you in the future, and keep you up to date with treatment options. Both of you have a responsibility to keep the channels open and the information flowing.

Any information you receive in a healthcare context can have an emotional effect. With medical problems we are often primed to expect bad news. This is certainly true when receiving a diagnosis, but it can also be the case during treatment and follow-up. It is not easy to receive disappointing news about your health but neither is it easy to give it, and some doctors do this better than others.

In the context of being a full participant in your healthcare decisions you need to be informed about your treatment options, and this can only happen if information is given to you in a relevant and meaningful way. There are two sides to this: when you receive information you must be open to it, and the person providing the information must be knowledgeable and sensitive to how it is likely to be received.

The following can be helpful in getting the most out of your consultation with medical professionals:

- Write down any questions you have in advance of your appointment. When you see the medical professional with a list to hand, it can help to jog your memory and keep you on track. Worry, fear, anxiety, side effects of medication and other factors may interfere with your recall and prevent you from getting the most out of your consultation. It is all too often the case that patients leave a consultation wondering why they forgot to ask a particular question which had been nagging at them.
- Take a notebook in which you can write down any information you are given (including the answers to your questions, of course). Appointments can feel stressful and rushed and it may be difficult to remember what has been said to you. Ask the medical

professional to write things down for you if you are unsure of being able to do it yourself for some reason (such as the spelling of medical terminology). A sketch about your condition and how it is affecting your body, a few bullet points to remind you about dietary restrictions or a numbered plan of your treatment schedule, made while you are hearing this information being given, can help you to recall what was said far more vividly than if you just try to recall it all from memory later on. Ask if there is any printed information you may take away with you.

- Consider taking someone else with you, not only for support but also as an extra pair of ears. Another person's presence in the consultation may help you to feel better understood, and you can then discuss the session later, which will help you to recall what was said and fix it more clearly in your mind. The other person may have comprehended something in a different way from you, and this will either help to deepen your understanding or raise a question that needs to be settled at your next consultation. When we are stressed and worried, we sometimes do not hear things in the way they were intended. What is said is not always what was meant or what we hear, and another pair of ears and another point of view can be invaluable. Complex dynamics are at play when there is a doctor–patient relationship; often, disturbing or upsetting things have to be said, so there is plenty of room for missed information or misunderstanding. You yourself may not actually want to hear some things – even though you have asked for the information ('Please tell me everything [but only if the news is good]'). The medical professional may collude with this by only giving partial information and not addressing all aspects of your concerns, and an outside eye may well pick up on this dynamic and be able to intervene.
- Do not feel disheartened if your medical professional appears somewhat impatient with you. Most medical professionals are busy and under constant pressure to complete detailed forms and keep clinical records. Increasingly today the use of a computer minimizes the amount of eye contact you have with a medical professional, and this can make the consultation feel impersonal. You will be one of many patients he or she sees and, essentially, to that person you are a clinical case. Also, trying to maintain a professional demeanour during the consultation can sometimes come across as being impersonal.
- If you feel unhappy with your care, try asking for more time or talk to the person who referred you, such as your GP. There is usually

a formal procedure for feedback and complaint in both the NHS and private clinics, and most hospitals have a Patient Advice and Liaison Service (PALS). The job of the PALS is to facilitate a good experience between you and your medical professionals.

- Do not be afraid to ask someone his or her name and role. It is likely that, particularly if you have a complex medical condition, you will meet a wide range of medical professionals and paramedic staff during your treatment and, of course, there is a hierarchy within each sphere ('Is this a consultant or the surgeon?' 'Is this a ward manager or a healthcare assistant?'). Hopefully, medical professionals will follow good practice, introducing themselves and explaining their role in your care and in the wider team. They may well also copy you into communications about your treatment and care.

The UK Department of Health has published a leaflet that aims to help people get the most out of their appointments. The suggestions in this leaflet are:

Before you leave your appointment, make sure you know the following:

- What is wrong? You might ask the following questions:

  'Can I check that I have understood what you've told me? What you've said is . . .'
  'Please would you explain it again? I don't understand.'
  'Please may I have a copy of any letters and so on written about me?'
  'Please would you draw a diagram showing me what you've just said?'

- What about further tests, such as blood tests, scans, etc.? You might ask the following questions:

  'What are the tests for?'
  'How and when will I get the results?'
  'Who should I contact if I don't get the results?'

- What treatment, if any, is best for you? You might ask the following questions:

  'Are there any ways to treat my condition?'
  'What do you recommend?'
  'Are there any side effects or risks to this treatment?'
  'For how long will I need treatment?'

'How effective is this treatment?'
'How will I know if the treatment is working?'
'What will happen if I don't have treatment?'
'Is there anything I should stop doing or avoid doing?'
'Is there anything I can do to help myself?'

- What happens next, and is there anyone you can contact for help? You might ask the following questions:

'What happens next – do I come back and see you?'
'Who do I contact if things get worse?'
'Do you have any printed information I can take away with me?'
'Where can I go for more information?'

For the full leaflet, see <www.nhs.uk/NHSEngland/AboutNHSservices/questionstoask/Pages/Makethemostofyourappointment.aspx>.

Receiving healthcare can sometimes be time-intensive. You may spend hours travelling to and from your doctor or hospital, waiting in queues, waiting for referrals and test results, and actually receiving treatment. This inevitable waiting can easily lead to further distress. Friends or family accompanying you to appointments can ease some of the burden and provide company and relief on these occasions.

Be proactive

It is never easy to face up to and manage the realities of living with a medical problem. If you can take a more active role in your self-management, you are likely to have a better outcome in the long run. Being proactive in the context of illness is about acknowledging that you have a responsibility for aspects of your own health and wellbeing, and about making an effort to influence your experience based on the choices available to you.

One way you can be proactive about your medical condition is to keep up to date with developments and new treatments. Some medical trials may affect your treatment; clinical trials and medical studies of new treatments may be relevant to your condition. Your doctor will almost certainly be aware of trials that are relevant to your condition, so you can discuss these together.

Ask for help

You do not need to deal with challenges on your own. In many cases, of course, it simply will not be possible for you to cope on your own.

It is important for you – for us all – to recognize when help is needed and to be able to ask for it.

There are several places you can turn to for help. What suits you will depend on your personality and your particular medical challenges. Side effects such as nausea, hair loss, bloating and weight gain, sleep disruption and skin reactions are usually temporary but can be particularly distressing. There are treatments available for many such side effects, and you should talk to your GP or other medical professional about these. With physical symptoms such as pain or fatigue your coping threshold may be more obvious to you, but with other challenges such as emotional difficulties it is harder to recognize when help is needed. The majority of people manage well on their own in the main and have no continuing issues, but how do you know when you need help with your emotional problems? What might prompt the involvement of medical professionals?

The following can give you an indication that emotional support is needed:

- experiencing the same issues repeatedly;
- feeling that you need a fresh perspective;
- needing help with a specific challenge (such as coping with pain, sexual problems or relationship difficulties);
- experiencing persistent and very intense emotions, such as overwhelming feelings of depression, loss or fear;
- needing to pre-empt problems, especially those associated with difficult times;
- worrying about relationships, particularly if you feel you are to blame for relationship problems with loved ones;
- promptings from other people: if people who care about you and know you well suggest that you need help with an emotional issue, it may be time to act on their advice.

What to expect from professional emotional support

Many medical specialisms integrate emotional support with medical treatment. This is most obvious in the treatment of cancer, infectious diseases (such as HIV disease), cardiac disease, diabetes and some dermatological conditions, and also in some other conditions such as chronic fatigue.

While professional mental health support might be suggested and should be readily available, this does not automatically mean that you have a serious mental health problem. Modern treatment centres recognize that receiving a diagnosis of a serious medical condition and coping with treatment can be stressful for you and your loved ones. The provision of mental healthcare is an option, should you need it. If it is not available in your clinic, you should ask your doctor to refer you to somewhere where it is. Failing this, your GP should have access to psychological support services within the practice.

There are different groups of mental health professionals who approach treatment of this type in different ways. Some explore experiences in your past and how these have impacted on the way you are coping now. Other approaches are very client-centred, where the professionals are empathetic listeners but offer little in the way of specific information or guidance – they enable you to feel heard in order that you can come up with your own solutions to your problems and issues. The approaches based on CBT involve working towards a solution in partnership with your therapist. This is a more scientific and rational approach to behaviour change, in line with the approach in this book. CBT may be short term or useful to you at different points or stages. Both CBT and mindfulness-based therapies aim to equip you with skills and strategies to enhance your coping and overall resilience.

Other mental health professionals focus specifically on helping people with couple or family relationship issues. Family and couples therapists may or may not have specialist knowledge of your medical condition, but will focus on the impact of illness on close relationships.

Counselling has different purposes, and the approach should reflect your needs. Some counsellors provide information, such as facts about your illness, advice about test results, prevention strategies, information about treatment options and drug trials, etc. This is particularly relevant when the psychological support of aspects of care is interwoven with the physical aspects of treatment, such as in oncology clinics. Other counsellors will discuss the implications of the information, such as any lifestyle changes needed to accommodate your treatment regimens. In supportive counselling the consequences – usually the emotional consequences – of the information are discussed. Psychotherapeutic counselling is more in depth and focuses on feeling, psychological adjustment, coping and problem resolution.

The authors of this book are experienced in several therapy approaches, and we use ideas and skills from them all interchangeably in our clinical work. We are often asked in medical clinics: 'How will

I know if my counsellor or psychologist or psychotherapist is helping me?' The simple answer is that if it feels as though your specific problem or concern is being addressed and feels less of a challenge after sessions, then your mental healthcare is probably working. If the focus of your sessions appears to have moved away from what is important to you, discuss your concern with your therapist. If you are not happy with where your therapy is going and feel that your concerns are not being addressed, it is probably time to look for another therapist.

Some people have the idea that counselling involves long-term commitment and regular appointments. This is sometimes the case, but not always. Increasingly, in healthcare settings such as the NHS it is unlikely that long-term psychological support will be provided. How often and over what period you see a psychologist or counsellor depends on what you want from the sessions, what your needs are and what resources are available, bearing in mind that there is high demand for psychologists and therapists in this type of setting.

Sometimes a single session can be sufficient, or intermittent sessions with a therapist as and when the need arises may be the best model for you. Or you may prefer regular sessions so you can be assured of a more constant external emotional support system. (This last may sometimes require accessing help privately, outside the NHS.)

A good therapist will work hard to understand you well, building on your strengths and working with you in your context to help you find a way to minimize the negative impact of your illness on your life.

As we have seen in this chapter, coping with a serious, complex or acute medical problem will engage you with healthcare professionals and health systems, and it is important that you feel comfortable with the people who are looking after you and treating you. It is equally important that you work in partnership with them to ensure that your care is relevant to your own circumstances and that communication with each medical professional feels open and useful.

It is also important that you take some responsibility for ensuring optimal outcomes in medical consultations. Stress, anxiety, low mood, side effects of medication and generally feeling unwell from your medical condition can all work against you in such contexts, as they may interfere with communication and sometimes leave you feeling dissatisfied with the consultation. Accordingly, prepare yourself for your consultations and seriously consider taking someone else with you to facilitate communication and your understanding of what happens.

A good, open and supportive relationship with your healthcare professionals is an important component of good coping.

10

How to support a friend, partner or family member who is unwell

It is not always easy for family members or friends to know exactly what they should do to help you. They may find it difficult to come to terms with the news of your condition, or they may feel unskilled or unprepared in helping you to cope. This chapter will show friends and relatives how to support someone who has been diagnosed with an acute or chronic condition.

When you learn that someone close has a serious health problem, you may initially feel overwhelmed and have no idea of what to do. Remember, though, that you are not alone, and that you are not the only one who can support the person who is unwell. Nor, perhaps, should you be. If you are not a qualified therapist or psychologist, it would be unreasonable to expect you to deliver 'therapy'. Do ask the medical team for what guidance you need – the team can also help you obtain further support, including a good counsellor, therapist or psychologist.

You may need to encourage your friend or relative to seek professional help. People's levels of distress may prevent them from taking the necessary steps to seek additional help. They may also feel embarrassed or ashamed of their poor health, and may be struggling with the uncertainty of not knowing exactly what the future holds.

Types of support

The exact nature of your support may depend upon the nature of the condition (as explored in Chapter 2), the preferences and wishes of the person who is unwell, the way she manages her own condition (or doesn't) and the nature of your relationship with her. Caring for someone who is confined to bed may be different from supporting someone with diabetes. Furthermore, a partner or a parent may be more subject to the daily impact of the physical condition than, for example, a colleague or an acquaintance. No two people are exactly the same, and it is therefore important to understand that no two people who are unwell will describe the same experience both on a physical and on an emotional level. This can be illustrated by considering the following two examples:

> Lilly, aged 30, had suffered from eczema and psoriasis since her early 20s. The eczema was particularly bad during periods of stress, often resulting in hospital admissions when her skin became infected. Lilly's parents tried their best to support her but they feared that they did not always get it right. They frequently invited her to stay with them in the family home, thinking that this would help reduce stress and therefore make her life easier. Lilly always declined, saying that she was not a baby any more and that she had to continue to live her life despite her condition. She would often get annoyed with her parents, feeling that they treated her like a child and did not really understand her needs as an independent woman. The parents were concerned that Lilly did not take their advice and felt that she was trying to 'put on a brave face'. Lilly, on the other hand, preferred to deal with her condition by not letting it ruin her life.

> Roger was diagnosed with severe rheumatoid arthritis, which led him to retire early from his job as a supervisor in a grocery store. His wife, Ellen, worked as a part-time librarian but took early retirement to support him. They had been married for 40 years, with three children and eight grandchildren. There were days when Roger was able to leave his bed and carry out light tasks around the house, but on those days when the pain was too intense, Ellen would make sure that he ate at least two meals a day and would spend most of her evening sitting by the side of his bed just chatting or reading to him. Roger felt an enormous sense of gratitude towards his wife and he often praised her kindness. Ellen knew that he would have done the same for her if things had been the other way around.

As we can see, different people may require differing support depending on their personality and the nature of their health problem. Lilly felt that it was important to maintain her independence, whereas her parents would have preferred to be more involved in her care. Roger and Ellen, on the other hand, felt that caring for a partner was the natural and obvious thing to do. This may work for some couples, while other couples may find it better to seek additional help from other family members or a professional.

There are three main kinds of support that family members can offer:

1 Practical support – such as help with mobility, doing the cooking and washing, assisting with visits to the doctor or clinic, and help with changing a dressing.
2 Financial support – including help with income and living expenses, going to work to make up the shortfall in loss of income due to the family member's inability to work, paying for prescription charges and paying for private healthcare.
3 Social and emotional support – being there and available to talk and listen, accompanying the person to a chemotherapy or treatment session, giving support and offering encouragement, making him or her laugh and at times offering a shoulder to cry on.

It may be neither possible nor appropriate for every family member to provide all three kinds of support. Instead, different family members might be better placed to offer some aspects of support than others. In particular, in some families where more than one person has a serious or chronic health problem (such as where one parent has cancer and the other has HIV infection, for example), it may be necessary to access support from outside the immediate family.

What role should I take?

Some people find it difficult to know exactly how they want others to support them. This may be because they are unsure themselves how they feel about their health and how their condition will affect their lives. Some people may find it unpleasant to think of their illness because they fear its consequences – losing their job, losing their former ability to function or even death. Others may feel too ashamed to talk about their health, or they may worry that they are burdening others by being unwell in the first place. For these reasons, when talking to your friend or relative, it is important to keep in mind that he or she may not feel able to talk about the illness or give you full details. It may therefore be helpful for both you and the person concerned to consider the following questions:

• How does the person feel about his or her illness?
• How do you feel about it?
• Does he or she want to talk about it? If so, when is a good time to do so?
• Are there any particular health-related topics that he or she does

not wish to discuss? Are there any immediate considerations that he or she prefers to talk about?

* Is there anyone else that should know about it (for example, children, extended family, other friends or colleagues)?
* What would be an appropriate way to tell others about your friend or family member's illness? When would be a good time to disclose this news?
* Are there any practical issues that need to be considered?

Do not be afraid to ask how he or she would like you to give support. We sometimes assume that we know what a partner, close friend or family member needs. This can lead to misunderstandings, even if our actions are carried out with the best intentions. One person, for example, may prefer to be accompanied during hospital visits; someone else, by contrast, may prefer to face a challenge alone or to have some physical distance from others when receiving treatment. What is useful for one individual may not necessarily be the same for another. You are more likely to be genuinely helpful if you and the person concerned work together to establish how much or how little you should be involved, and how best to react when he or she is actively symptomatic or receiving treatment.

> Iman's best friend, Paul, had a stroke six weeks ago, which left him paralysed on the whole of the left side of his body. Paul has recently been discharged from the intensive care unit and is undergoing long-term rehabilitation to learn to walk again. Iman tries to visit Paul as often as he can but has sometimes felt unsure as to how much or how little he should talk about Paul's health. During one visit, Paul mentioned how much he appreciated Iman's support. Iman thought that this was a good time to talk to Paul about how he could best support him. This led to a constructive conversation about the fact that Paul wants Iman first and foremost to be his friend, someone he can discuss football and sport with rather than have deep conversations about his feelings. Paul told Iman that he is seeing a therapist twice a week as part of the rehabilitation programme.

There is a great deal of information in books and online about various conditions, both acute/serious and chronic. Take the time to learn as much as you can better to understand the nature of the condition, how it manifests and how it can impact on a person's life, family and friends. This can be a helpful way of letting someone know that you are interested in his or her illness and that you want to give support in the best way you can. As we have already stated, positive, encouraging and supportive behaviours can help to remove or relieve feelings of shame or embarrassment, loneliness and anxiety, which can in itself be therapeutic.

Tips for providing social and emotional support

Here are some suggestions that you may wish to consider when supporting a partner, parent, child or friend who has an illness:

- Take the time to listen to the other person's thoughts and feelings about the condition. Sometimes he or she will just want someone to talk to, and by offering the time and space where concerns can be processed you are likely to provide enormous support.
- Be empathetic towards your friend's situation. Try to imagine what it feels like.
- Don't be afraid to ask questions. This can often show the other person that you are listening to his or her concerns, that you are interested in the condition and that you are there to provide support.
- Don't assume that you should be able to offer a solution to the problem. Instead, try to visualize yourself as a supportive shoulder to lean on, someone who is there when your friend needs to talk or requires help with practical matters.
- You may also want to help the person re-establish the sense of a normal life. This could be achieved by taking the initiative to resume some of your shared activities, if possible, such as going to the cinema, watching a rugby game together, going for a walk and so on.
- Be respectful towards the other person's preferences, wishes and needs. This is especially important when it concerns issues surrounding the illness.
- Try to keep an open communication whenever possible. Ask: 'How would you like me to support you?' 'Is there anything in particular you want me to do?' 'Is there anything I am doing that I could do differently?' 'How and when is a good time to talk about the way we communicate with each other?'

Supporting you as a helper

Another important thing to consider is that the effects of health problems can at times be as challenging to a partner, family member or friend as they are to the person who is ill. It is important also to consider support for yourself, as how you cope is likely to influence how the unwell person copes, and vice versa. When it comes to coping with issues surrounding illness, or indeed with most other forms of psychological difficulty, the state of our family relationships, as well as how our partners or close friends adapt to the situation, may matter more to us than anything else. Where close relationships come to feel tense, strained, emotionally distant or volatile, these changes can tip the balance and make us susceptible to increased anxiety, depression and hopelessness. An understanding of how relationships can be affected paves the way for more open communication and improved support, both of which have been linked to more favourable health outcomes.

Here are some tips on how you can take care of yourself while supporting a friend or a family member who is unwell:

- Do you have anyone you can talk to about your own feelings? It may be helpful to talk to other family members, colleagues or friends.
- Keeping a reflective diary to express your emotions, thoughts and ideas can also be very helpful.
- You may want to ask around to see if there is a support group for friends, family members and carers that you could attend.
- Although your life may have been affected by a close family member or friend's condition, it is important that you try to continue with regular activities. This can help to establish a sense of normality.
- You are likely to feel worried or stressed by the situation. Physical exercise, yoga, relaxation and any other activities that help you to feel relaxed can help to combat stress.
- Don't be afraid to seek professional support, such as speaking to the medical team to obtain information, or to consider seeing a counsellor, therapist or psychologist to help you process the situation.

For most people, family and friends are the most important source of support in the face of illness. A good way to support someone who is unwell is not to be afraid to ask how he or she wants to be supported. Other ways include offering open communication, active and empathetic listening and showing the other person that you are interested in the health problem. However, others within the family can experience intense emotional reactions on being told of the illness. It is therefore important that you as a supporter take care of yourself. There is some truth in the saying that 'you can't take care of someone else unless you are OK yourself'.

11

What to do
if this book is not enough

This chapter addresses why sometimes progress may be slower than you had hoped or expected, and what you can do. We have included it as we recognize that some people might need more help than this book can provide. This chapter is also designed to reassure you that it is entirely normal to feel that you have not overcome all your unwelcome emotions if or when you find them recurring. As we have mentioned, feelings engendered by medical problems tend to wax and wane, because of many varying factors.

Most of what we have covered in this book addresses self-help strategies, skills and techniques to help you to understand and begin to overcome the main psychological effects of living with illness or other physical health issues.

We hope that this book has helped you gain a better understanding of some of the more common psychological reactions to living with medical problems, and how health conditions can affect our relationships with our loved ones. Chapter 9 shed light on relationships with professional caregivers, and this is equally important when we consider how illness affects us emotionally, in that communication with professional caregivers needs to be optimized, if you are to feel confident and supported by them.

You may already have had the chance to reflect on and try out some of the ideas in this book. As we said right at the beginning, there is no single 'one-size-fits-all' solution to the complex issues that arise in the context of serious and chronic health conditions. People react differently to different diagnoses, and their reaction will depend on their stage of life, the nature of their condition, the support they have around them, and many other factors we have highlighted throughout this book. Different approaches and solutions need to be tried out in order to discover which works best for you. It is a form of trial and error, but since everything we have described in this book is based on tried-and-tested, well-researched techniques, there will be at least some which are effective for you.

If you have gained insight into how being unwell can lead to feelings of depression and anxiety but do not yet feel sufficiently confident to apply some of the techniques we have described, do not despair. Recognizing the connection between medical events as they affect you and your emotional reactions to them is an important starting point, and it is sometimes only over a period of time that the right key to fit the lock is found. You might need time, persistence and patience. Coping emotionally with medical problems is seldom a clear-cut and definable objective. Simply because you are able to overcome stress, anxiety, low mood and other psychological reactions does not mean that you are content with the challenges of illness, or ready to accept them. Indeed, coping with the emotional side of the challenge is only one aspect of overall coping. As much as we would like to promote the goal of psychological therapy as being no more depression, anxiety or emotional distress, in fact therapy is not likely to be the whole answer. You may be able to cope well with some of these negative feelings for periods of time but, due to the changing course of your illness, shifting patterns of support from your loved ones and/or professionals or many other factors, at other times you may be less able to cope. It is fair to say that, for many people living with chronic health conditions, a relapsing–remitting reaction is the norm rather than the exception. There may be good days and bad, periods when you are on top of life and periods when life feels overwhelming. The ideas in this book should provide you with the signposts and coping skills for when the negative feelings return.

Being able to share your feelings with family members, friends, work colleagues and others, as well as medical professionals, is an important starting point for coping more successfully with emotional problems. In most areas of our lives, sharing problems with others has the effect of diminishing the intensity and fear we suffer in relation to a challenge. The old saying 'A problem shared is a problem halved' holds very true in relation to the topics covered in this book.

As psychologists, we understand that speaking to others about feelings may, in itself, be challenging. In our experience the process of talking to other people can put someone in a catch-22 situation: on the one hand, as we have discussed, talking to others can make us feel connected and less frightened by what we face; on the other hand we may worry about burdening our friends and loved ones, or about seeming weak or lacking in coping skills or resilience by opening up to others.

Talking to other people about how we feel is often no easy feat. If you are not used to doing this, or have taken particular pride in having managed most of your personal difficulties and challenges without having to turn to others for help, the challenge of now having to do so can be particularly hard.

Some reasons why progress may be slow

This section lists some of the more common explanations of why you might continue to experience anxiety and depression despite your efforts. This is by no means an exhaustive or complete list, but you can use it as a checklist to measure your own progress and evaluate any continuing difficulties. Having some understanding of why you are continuing to struggle with strong and unwelcome emotions should enable you to gain a deeper understanding of how being unwell affects you, and how more specialist psychological help can assist at this time.

Working too hard at solutions

You may well be familiar with the half-humorous definition of insanity (often attributed to Einstein): 'Doing the same thing over and over again and expecting different results'. This can be applied to most psychological difficulties, and coping with medical problems is no exception. If, for example, your attempted solution to anxiety is to undertake relaxation exercises and increase physical activity as a way of releasing endorphins into your bloodstream to raise your mood, you may find this difficult to implement if, for example, your medical condition prevents you from undertaking regular aerobic exercise. Your progress may also be hijacked if medication you have been prescribed actually increases anxiety. One example of this is people undergoing chemotherapy for certain cancers, where steroids might be prescribed: as many patients complain, a side effect of this medication is that it causes raised heart rate, makes you feel sweaty and agitated and interferes with sleep.

Sometimes, too, people avoid acting on solutions, as it all seems to be too much hard work. You might be at a low ebb and feel depleted physically, which may make active problem-solving seem just too hard.

Do not worry if, in the first instance, your natural reaction is avoidance. It is not essential to try and overcome all your difficult feelings immediately. Indeed, as psychologists we would argue that it is not necessarily a requirement that someone living with a chronic health condition should be entirely free of unpleasant emotions. It is part of life that, when we are faced with challenges and adversity, we react quite normally in ways that reflect psychological distress, and our emotions can be a sign of this. Low mood may be a consequence of feeling challenged; anxiety may arise because we feel out of control or are worrying about an outcome. The feelings themselves are not the problem; it is the effect they have on you and how you respond to them which is sometimes the problem. Therefore we need to develop methods and techniques for curtailing and reducing the escalation of feelings and your responses to them.

As we have pointed out before in this book, there is a wide range of cognitive and behavioural techniques, skills and interventions you can use in order to challenge and overcome anxiety and depression and other emotional difficulties. However, if you avoid situations where you can try out the effectiveness of these and measure your progress, they will remain merely textbook ideas. At some point you need to move the ideas from the page into the real world and test how they work for you. This can sometimes be daunting or stressful, or even feel emotionally too painful. If this is the case, then you may need to go back a step or two so that you are not overwhelmed by your feelings.

With most psychological difficulties it is preferable to take gradual, comfortable-but-determined steps forward and to gain confidence as you go, rather than taking giant leaps and risking everything. There is little point in escalating stress and anxiety to levels that feel unbearable. It may be necessary to try something else, or something less difficult. For example, if you tried to challenge some of your negative automatic thoughts but found yourself upset, tearful and unable even to challenge any of your thoughts, ending up even more stressed than when you started the exercise, then perhaps you attempted too big a first step. Once you have taken time out and calmed down, reflected and perhaps talked it over with someone who understands what you are going through, it may be worth scaling your next interventions back, initially just to listing some of the feelings you have experienced in the previous 24 hours. Just measuring and noting your feelings, looking at patterns of when they occur, seeing if there are times of the day when you experience them more, and examining the specific nature of the feelings (similar to keeping a mood diary) can be a useful starting point. Remind yourself that scaling back in this way does not mean that you have 'failed' – you have had the courage to try to take a large step forward. It may have been initially too challenging and so made you anxious, but you will still almost certainly have learned something in the process. Gaining confidence with small steps is arguably better than taking giant leaps which are likely to expose you to greater stress and anxiety, and potentially put you off even making the attempt in future.

If your thoughts about what you need to do leave you feeling emotionally vulnerable and upset, then perhaps it is time to go back to gaining a clear understanding of these thoughts and explore your fundamental fear about what you think may happen to you. It may be that your underlying fear of something catastrophic happening (such as dying or your incapacitation increasing) is what is driving your anxiety and low mood. This may need further exploration and attention and itself may need to be a target of intervention. We would recommend that, in this case, you speak to a trusted friend, or to a psychologist or therapist who specializes in working with health-related problems.

Being able to work on these difficulties now

Motivational issues can also interfere with progress in psychological therapy generally. This is not to suggest that people who have psychological issues relating to health problems do not wish to overcome them – most of the time this is not the case. However, it is not always possible to give the time, focus and intensity needed in order to overcome the difficulties sufficiently. This might be because you are stressed or are facing other difficulties in your life that are distracting you from dealing with the matter in hand. Facing up to difficulties is rarely something we do independently from other issues in our lives. It might be that you are having a difficult time at work, for example, or are stressed by a child playing up or are facing financial difficulties. Health problems rarely present on their own or in a vacuum, and they are usually a further challenge in an already complex and challenged life. Furthermore, as we have emphasized previously, the nature of your condition, the side effects of treatment, the emotional impact of what you are going through, among many other factors, may also be weighing down on you and making it difficult to rise to the challenge and work clearly and methodically towards overcoming your psychological issues around your illness.

Motivation may also be affected by living with anxiety and depression over a long period of time. The effect of this can be that you have experienced reasonable coping and have found ways of avoiding or managing the anxiety and depression rather than confronting them. Sometimes being comfortable with our own solution to a difficulty, even though it is not a total solution, can interfere with our efforts to overcome and cure the difficulty in the long run.

Motivational issues are also relevant in respect of the effort required. There is hardly any psychological issue or emotional reaction to being unwell that does not require some effort to overcome it. This is no different from gaining new skills in other areas of life. Do you remember when you learned how to use a computer or learned to drive? In psychological therapy, the initial stages can feel awkward, stressful and difficult. If you are struggling, it may be helpful to reflect on your original motivation to overcome your difficulties. It is also essential to identify whether there are other factors, such as the nature of your health condition, the specific symptoms it engenders, side effects of medication and other factors that may be interfering with your motivation.

If you find that your efforts on your own are insufficient, it is probably sensible to seek help by consulting a psychologist or therapist. Many have extensive experience of working with people who have health-related problems and will understand much of your experience. They will also appreciate that the impact of this type of problem extends beyond you as an individual and will be aware of the ripple effect it can have on people who are close to you.

From time to time a doctor may also recommend that you take medication in order to help speed up the process of overcoming some of the difficult feelings you may be experiencing. There is a well-recognized link between continuing and intense feelings of anxiety and depression and physical health outcomes, and your doctor would not want you to become any more unwell as a result of the psychological distress you experience. Modern medications for anxiety and depression are on the whole safe and effective; they do not cause dependency and have minimal side effects. Medical treatment of mood difficulties is a specialist area that may involve seeking the opinion of a psychiatrist in order to ensure that the most appropriate medication is prescribed for you.

Am I using the right 'new' solution for me?

It can be that the new solution you are applying is still not the best one for you. If, for example, you try to challenge negative automatic thoughts but fail to back this up with complementary behavioural changes, your progress is likely to be limited or temporary. Conversely, if you change some of your behaviour without changes in your thoughts about anxiety and depression, your progress may also be curtailed. We have deliberately highlighted a range of different approaches rather than single, stand-alone ones. Choosing only one may simply not be enough – it may be necessary to identify and apply several to improve your general psychological wellbeing. Think of it as multifaceted rather than a single challenge.

It may also be useful to identify specific situations in which negative feelings are most likely. Increased anxiety, for example, is common before medical check-ups, X-rays or scans, or before surgery. It may be worth targeting events that cause the most distress to you (or your loved ones), particularly if they become recurrent features of your care.

What else is happening in your life now?

Psychological difficulties, as we have said, rarely exist in total isolation from other issues in our lives. We have particularly addressed this point above, but it is worth stressing here that there may be what are termed 'cofactors' that interfere with your progress or maintain some of the unwelcome feelings you may be experiencing. If you are experiencing low mood or have a condition such as acne, a nervous twitch, blushing for a medical reason and suchlike which affects your behaviour or appearance, this additional issue may have an impact on how you cope with the more chronic and serious condition. Addressing your anxiety and depression without first taking into account these additional issues or cofactors may slow down your progress.

This is not to say that an individual who has acne needs to be completely free from the condition or that a person with depression should be in perfect psychological shape before attending to his or her low mood following a heart attack. What it does mean is that cofactors like these should be taken into account when coming to understand your emotional response to your medical condition.

What is success?

Setting your sights on an instant and total cure for anxiety and depression in the face of illness may be a bridge too far. Experience tells us that the treatment of anxiety and depression can take time and progress may be gradual and incremental. Furthermore, if you have a lifelong medical condition, the unwelcome and difficult feelings around this do not go away for all time just because you have successfully treated them on one particular occasion. They are likely to return at various points, and this is normal. It is a reflection of being human that we respond differently to situations at different times in our lives. If you follow these standard psychological methods, using CBT and mindfulness as described in this book, you can expect progress to be gradual – sometimes a touch slow, but nevertheless incremental.

Treatment, whether with a psychologist, therapist or counsellor or through self-help, requires time, patience, perseverance and a measure of determination. There may be occasional setbacks, or at times it may feel as if you are playing a game of snakes and ladders. It can feel as if progress has been suddenly reversed, but then it quickly picks up steam again. Maintaining a positive outlook, having a healthy dose of motivation and keeping in mind the ideas described in this book will help you to keep focused and on track.

When you set goals, it is important to make sure they are appropriate and realistic for you. It is easy to set unachievable and unhelpful goals. This usually ends in failure, which can then make you feel despondent and less motivated. A helpful model is the 'SMART' goals model. SMART stands for:

Specific – make a goal as specific as possible.
Measurable – make sure that the goal can be measured.
Achievable – is your goal achievable in the next couple of weeks?
   (If not, then you might want to break it down into smaller and shorter-term goals.)
Relevant – make sure that this goal is important to you and that you are aware of the benefits that would come with achieving it.
Time-specific – it is helpful to set a time frame in which you want to achieve the goal.

Getting the right support

Involving others in your treatment and problem-solving can be enormously helpful. We do recognize, however, that for some people this is especially difficult. You may find it embarrassing or stressful, or feel it gives others the impression that you are not coping, so triggering alarm bells in them and perhaps leading to their being over-concerned or emotionally smothering.

Obviously we would encourage you to share your feelings in conversation. In our experience, trained professionals have already encountered many people with similar difficulties, so it will be neither new nor uncomfortable to them. On the contrary, it is their job to help you with such difficulties, and they should provide you with every encouragement along the way. Most psychological problems and difficulties are treatable.

Your starting point of discussion with a professional, if you decide to seek such help, could be this book, which may have highlighted some of the difficulties you might be experiencing. You could perhaps describe any techniques you have tried and any limitations you have come up against. This is a useful starting point for discussion.

We recognize that taking the issue to someone else means facing up to it and verbalizing it, which is a step in itself. Think of it as part of the therapeutic process. Describing the difficulty and talking about it with another person is almost always, in itself, beneficial. If anyone is judgemental, dogmatic, closed-minded, indifferent or simply does not have the time to listen to you – whether that person is a friend, family member or (hopefully not) a professional – stop talking to them! It will inevitably leave you feeling much worse if you try to talk to someone who makes you feel shut out or shows no interested in listening to you.

A session with your GP, psychologist, counsellor or therapist will help to put you back on track by assessing the nature and extent of your anxiety and depression and how best to treat it. This book can then act as a companion to the face-to-face treatment. You can use it to help you think about homework exercises and to plot your progress in overcoming anxiety, depression and other emotional difficulties.

If you have not made all the progress you would like

If you have decided that it is too difficult for you to act on the ideas suggested in this book at this time, or you have made some progress but feel it is not enough, you may become over-critical of yourself. You might feel a sense of failure for not having 'cured' your anxiety or depression. If you have worked through this book, it is likely that you have already made some progress, even if it is just in gaining an understanding of why you are feeling as you do. You should, at the very least, give yourself credit for having achieved this much.

Reading parts of this book means that you have shown the courage and motivation to take steps to understand and to overcome your emotional difficulties. As we have stressed throughout the book, these difficulties are normal and experiencing them, although unwelcome and at times very unpleasant, does not suggest that there is something mentally wrong with you. However, as we have also stressed, the effect that these difficulties have on your life, and their persistence and intensity, is something that you can improve.

References

1 Hofmann, S. G., Sawyer, A. T., Will, A. A. and Oh, D. (2010) 'The effects of mindfulness-based therapy on anxiety and depression: a meta-analytic review', *Journal of Consulting and Clinical Psychology*, 78 (2): 169–83.
2 Burch, V. and Penman, D. (2013) *Mindfulness for Health: A practical guide to relieving pain, reducing stress and restoring wellbeing*, London: Piatkus.

Further reading

Mindfulness

Burch, V. and Penman, D. (2013) *Mindfulness for Health: A practical guide to relieving pain, reducing stress and restoring wellbeing*, London: Piatkus.

Kabat-Zinn, Jon (2010) *Mindfulness Meditation for Pain Relief*, Louisville, Colorado, USA: Sounds True Inc. (audio CD).

Williams, M. and Penman, D. (2011) *Mindfulness: Finding peace in a frantic world*, London: Piatkus.

Cognitive behavioural therapy

Bor, Robert, Eriksen, Carina and Chaudry, Sara (2014) *Overcoming Stress*, London: Sheldon Press.

Burgess, Mary and Chalder, Trudie (2009) *Overcoming Chronic Fatigue: A self-help guide using cognitive behavioural techniques*, London: Robinson.

Cole, F., Howden-Leach, H., MacDonald, H. and Carus, C. (2005) *Overcoming Chronic Pain: A self-help guide using cognitive behavioural techniques*, London: Robinson.

Eriksen, Carina, Bor, Robert and Oakes, Margaret (2010) *The Panic Workbook*, London: Sheldon Press.

Espie, Colin (2006) *Overcoming Insomnia and Sleep Problems: A self-help guide using cognitive behavioural techniques*, London: Robinson.

Fennell, Melanie (2009) *Overcoming Low Self-esteem: A self-help guide using cognitive behavioural techniques*, London: Robinson.

Gilbert, Paul (2009) *Overcoming Depression: A self-help guide using cognitive behavioural techniques*, third edition, London: Robinson.

Gonzalez, Virginia (2010) *Living a Healthy Life with Chronic Conditions: Self-management of heart disease, arthritis, diabetes, asthma, bronchitis, emphysema and others*, Boulder, Colorado, USA: Bull Publishing.

Kennerley, Helen (2009) *Overcoming Anxiety: A self-help guide using cognitive behavioural techniques*, London: Robinson.

Lee, Deborah (2012) *The Compassionate Mind Approach to Recovering from Trauma Using Compassion Focused Therapy*, London: Robinson.

Veale, David and Willson, Rob (2009) *Overcoming Health Anxiety: A self-help guide using cognitive behavioural techniques*, London: Robinson.

Veale, David, Willson, Rob and Clarke, Alex (2009) *Overcoming Body Image Problems Including Body Dysmorphic Disorder: A self-help guide using cognitive behavioral techniques*, New York: Basic Books.

Williams, Chris (2011) *Overcoming Functional Neurological Symptoms: A five areas approach*, London: CRC Press.

Index